GENERAL EDITOR Edward Goldsmith

PROSPECT
FOR
MAN

'*Quant à la destinée
humaine pessimiste,
je suis optimiste
quant à l'Homme.*'—
ALBERT CAMUS

Living Dangerously

Living Dangerously

Hilda Cherry Hills

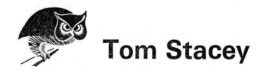 **Tom Stacey**

To Lawrence

Who walks beside me

First published in 1973
by Tom Stacey Ltd.,
28–29 Maiden Lane, London WC2E 7JP

Copyright © Hilda Cherry Hills 1973

ISBN 0 85468 406 9

Printed in Great Britain
by Richard Clay (The Chaucer Press) Ltd.,
Bungay, Suffolk

'Dangers by being despised grow great.'
EDMUND BURKE (1729–1797)

'I have milked a thousand cows, but the cheese is my own.'
CHARLES READE (1814–1884)

CONTENTS

FOREWORD   9

1   Air Pollution in the Home   11

2   Clearing the Air   35

3   Pollution in the Car   44

4   Tobacco—The Personal Pollution   55

5   The Importance of Being Parents   71

6   Danger. Women at Work   95

7   Insecticides Indoors   111

8   Alcoholism—Hidden Danger
to Health and Happiness   124

9   The Sweet Life   142

10   Fatness or Fitness?   156

11   Food Defences against Cancer   168

12   The Significance of Quality
in Food   186

13   Good Cooks and Good Health   197

14   The Need to 'have a Concern'   210

INDEX   216

Foreword

I have written this book to try to save lives, needless suffering and disability. Everyday life does not lack open and obvious dangers, but domestic perils are hidden, insidious and largely unsuspected by the majority who suffer the consequences while remaining unconscious of the causes.

We all need to become aware of these dangers and, even more important, we need to take action against them ourselves if life is to be lived at its best. Warnings are worthless unless they can lead to action, and the counter measures I suggest are all within our choice as individuals.

I am deeply grateful to the many authors writing in medical and other scientific journals and books from whose reports I have selected the facts on which this book is built. Those writing in French, Spanish and Italian I have translated myself. For those in German I am indebted for translations to Mrs K. Smith-Reitzner and Mrs Tamarkin, and for those in Russian to Mr John Perfect. I am further indebted to Miss E. Stevens, Librarian, Braintree, and to Mr J. Lace, County Librarian, Chelmsford, for making these many texts available.

My deepest gratitude goes to my husband, Lawrence Hills, for his forbearance and his frequently expressed doubts whether this book would ever reach completion, which have driven me doggedly to the end.

HILDA CHERRY HILLS

Cape Town, October 1960
Bocking, January 1971

1

Air Pollution in the Home

'The stryker with a knife under the cloke.'
                                    GEOFFREY CHAUCER

Most of us spend the greater part of our lives in some sort
of building. It is obviously of extreme importance that this most
intimate air should be kept free of harmful gases, while the oxygen
it normally contains should be treasured as a life-enhancing jewel
more precious than any diamond. Unfortunately few realize this
importance.

Life without either carbon or oxygen is inconceivable, but they
become a threat to life when combined in the act of burning to form
carbon monoxide, known to the chemist as CO. Carbon monoxide
is a killer. We all know that today. Then why do we allow it to
frequent our homes, polluting the air, robbing us of essential oxygen
and slowly eroding our health, for as J. B. S. Haldane has said, 'Not
only does CO stop the human machine, but it deteriorates the
machinery'? Where does this domestic CO come from?

The answer lies in the chemistry of combustion. When any substance whatever is burned, the products of its incomplete combustion,
which give out heat, light and energy, must contain CO from the
combination of the burning carbon with the oxygen in which alone it
can burn. Herein lies the danger, especially in enclosed places. The
source of harmful fumes need not even be some sort of fuel. This is
well illustrated in a medical report on some Italian workers who
suffered from CO intoxication caused by burning the potato chips
they were cooking on two occasions during cloudy weather, when the
ventilation system proved inefficient, and scanty dispersal of the
fumes built up a high CO content in the air in which they were
working.[1]

While oxygen free in air is one of the main pillars of life, when
combined with carbon in the form of carbon monoxide it becomes
not only a potential source of death but a constant dispenser of

12 Living Dangerously

discomfort and ill health. In fact, with the notable exception of electricity and nuclear energy, all our ways and systems of producing heat, light or energy indoors, for no matter what purpose, give out in some degree this dangerous gas, to pollute and in one sense poison the surrounding air.

It has been estimated that about one half of the two to three million tons of smoke* produced each year in Great Britain comes from domestic users. This smoke is a measure of incomplete combustion which releases not only CO but other noxious gases and particular elements into the domestic as well as the open air.

Smokeless but not fumeless
A scarcity of coke feared in the winter of 1968–9 forced the National Coal Board to drop one of its advertising campaigns. This may have been a useful factor in reducing cases of respiratory and other disabilities by preventing a number of households from banking up living-room fires with this fume-producing fuel. Why should survivors of winter trench warfare need reminding of the disabling and often lethal effects of burning coke in enclosed places; or those old enough to recall them, that night watchmen huddled in greatcoats were always careful to keep their braziers outside their open-ended huts? It has also been remarked by survivors of POW camps that men driven by the excessive cold at night to leave their bunks and lie down beside the burning braziers of bunk-houses failed to survive this practice for long. How is it that men's memories are so short?

The Post Office Engineering Research Station at Dollis Hill, London NW2, has an automatic apparatus for measuring hydrogen sulphide. This impurity in domestic gas is extremely toxic, and, with its equally unpleasant derivative sulphur dioxide (SO_2), is also produced by coke and fuel oil, contributing significantly to atmospheric pollution. On an average wintry day the amount registered is 0·05 ppm to 5 ppm, but on 6 December 1963 this rose at 6 pm to 35 ppm and fell again four days later to 0·25 ppm. Obviously, air recognizes no frontiers. If we or our neighbours put in oil or solid-fuel-fired central heating with a boiler chimney lower than the other chimney in the house or the higher parts of the road, these fumes will come in at doors and windows and blow down chimneys in heavily overcast or gusty weather. They can even come down fairly

* Unfortunately removing the smoke from a fuel does not prevent it producing other noxious fumes when in use.

tall chimneys, causing a suction on the lee side of the house or in some unlit chimney which can suck in a great deal. All this can take place in a smokeless zone, using smokeless fuel.

Volcanoes have been responsible for emitting sulphur dioxide (SO_2) vapours since before recorded time, and plants have learned to develop a defence against them and can convert sulphur dioxide to a harmless sulphate. Humans have not learned this useful trick, and seem unlikely to do so. Yet there are no clauses in the Clean Air Act restricting its domestic emission, though there are minimum heights specified for chimneys that emit large amounts. An economist and statistician, Mr Alan Smith, in a report which is unfortunately not likely to reach a wide public owing to its very high price, has presented many important proposals on this aspect of smokeless but not fumeless fuels. After congratulating the nation on its unique air pollution controls operated under the hundred-year-old Alkali Act, he stresses that a major attack must now be made on domestic air pollution. Though commending the National Coal Board and others on the production of smokeless fuels, he points out that 'in the long run, however, the use of such fuels should be discouraged, since they give rise to sulphur dioxide emission'.[2]

This SO_2 is produced whenever coal is burned and although wood, paraffin, and town or natural gas are relatively free, coke and anthracite still contain it. Yet, since both these have been officially blessed for use in a smokeless zone, the average person happily uses them to stoke up a daytime or all-night grate, boiler or cooker, apparently unaware that the invisible CO and SO_2 which a poorly drawing chimney, or a change in the wind or foggy or still conditions can produce, is a danger to health and even to life. SO_2 is both an irritant and a poison, and is so highly corrosive that it will, in time, completely ruin the chrome reflector of an electric heater in the same room. These potentially fatal fumes need not even be in the same room to do their deadly work, as is illustrated by the case of four young brothers who were found dead in bed by their parents, having been killed by the fumes from an all-night coke-burning boiler in the living-room below their bedroom. Two years later, in the summer of 1968, there were four deaths at different addresses in London, because the heat and humidity (the temperature stood at 90°F at the time) had caused fumes to block the chimneys of coke boilers used for hot water heating, so that fumes had seeped back along connecting chimneys into the rooms where they slept, presumably with open windows. Another victim had died from the same cause a few months earlier and this could hardly be blamed on the heat, since it occurred in March. The coroner's comment that these cases show that 'there is a very, very narrow margin between safety and extreme danger with these coke boilers' appeared to have attracted little attention.

Solid fuel cookers, heaters or hot water systems share the drawbacks of coke, and their presence cannot fail to be detected by sensitive nostrils immediately on entry into a house, though many owners seem oblivious to fumes which may be all too apparent to guests in whom they cause headaches and insomnia. This is underlined by a report from Holland dealing with indoor air pollution in Rotterdam in 1965. Eight hundred paired samples of air from sixty homes were studied. One home had a modern anthracite heater, and showed an indoor air concentration of sulphur dioxide, as compared with that outdoors, as below:

Date	SO_2 indoors	SO_2 outdoors
12 Feb.	1250	200
13 Feb.	782	197
14 Feb.	985	513
17 Feb.	776	195
18 Feb.	904	117
19 Feb.	623	190

The investigators point out: 'If one in a hundred houses has a faulty chimney or stove, one begins to wonder how far indoor concentrations of air pollution play a role in causing premature deaths in persons with failing circulation and respiration, and what role CO also plays in this process,' and surmise that 'faulty chimneys and heaters may play a bigger role in air pollution during fogs than has so far been suspected'.[3]

As well as being responsible for deaths, SO_2 contributes to bronchitis. A study of seven healthy men breathing it in by nose implied that chemically minute amounts reaching the larynx and lower airways is sufficient to set off reflex changes in bronchial tone.[4]

Appliances complacently considered efficient but in fact faulty, may be causing air pollution indoors whether there is a fog or not, especially if there are unfavourable weather conditions affecting downdraughts.

The menace of carbon monoxide

Carbon monoxide is loosely referred to as a poison. In fact it does not poison the body but starves it of essential oxygen. It is not a Borgia but a bandit, behaving like a murderously inclined robber, snatching away this most precious element as it courses on its way in the blood stream. This can be pictured as a stream of weak-tea coloured fluid flowing like a conveyor belt laden with sealed packets of red blood cells, each with its unique life-enhancing gift of haemoglobin-wrapped oxygen to be delivered to every one of our tissues and cells, whose number is astronomical. If we are breathing in CO these treasures never reach their goal, for CO has, in the language of the chemist, an affinity for the haemoglobin which is roughly 300 times as strong as the affinity of oxygen. This enables it to oust the oxygen from its place in as many of the packets as it can attack, and the blood flows on its course now carrying the compound called carboxyhaemoglobin in place of the oxygen which the cells require. Since they are unable to make use of the CO, they reject it, and the haemoglobin passes along with its cargo undelivered, and so back through the veins where the blood now looks as red as arterial blood, so that anyone suffering from a heavy dose of CO wears a permanent cherry-red blush on neck, face and extremities. Small amounts of CO, which supplant smaller amounts of oxygen, cause similar symptoms to those noted in anyone going up to high altitudes until their blood cells increase in number.

Breathing air containing 0·07 per cent or 7 ppm of CO ultimately converts about half the total haemoglobin, which carries the oxygen in the blood stream, into carboxyhaemoglobin, which is incapable of carrying any oxygen. An average man in normal health could just about survive this amount, with its consequent deterioration in his oxygen intake. It should be emphasized that while we may consume small quantities of poisons in food and drink, we eat only three or four times daily, but we breathe sixteen times per minute for twenty-four hours every day.*

Owing to these vast quantities of air we draw into our bodies, a very large dose of any air pollutant can be absorbed, even though it is only present in minute amounts in the air being breathed. But there is no unanimity of response to this invader.

A classic example of the enormous variability of reaction is that

* In one year an adult breathes 7,884,000 pints of air according to an editorial in the *British Medical Journal*, 15 October 1955.

given by the poisons expert, Gustav Schenk. Two men were unwittingly subjected to CO in a closed room. One man died at once, the other was only slightly ill.

The differing effects on different individuals of a sudden shortage of oxygen owing to a rapid rise in altitude is illustrated by an incident occurring in France in the 1870s. Three French scientists went up in a balloon. At 25,000 feet they all lost consciousness. Later one of them came to, to find they were descending safely with his companions still unconscious. His judgement impaired by his oxygen deficiency, he threw out more ballast. Up they rose, and once more he passed out. When he came round again about an hour later, the balloon was dropping rapidly and he was safe. But his companions were both dead.

Differing susceptibilities to CO in bodily systems
One reason for the wide range of disabilities arising from lack of oxygen is the varied part it plays in the different functions of the body. This role begins not at birth, as commonly supposed, but very soon after conception, and it accompanies us to the last second of our lives.

Oscar Wilde's quip when asked if life was worth living that 'That depends on the liver' might well be applied to the question why people react so variously to the same amount of CO in the air. Since liver cells are especially susceptible to deprivation of oxygen,[5] those with any kind of liver disability or malfunction from such factors as hepatitis (once so common before the issue of regulations ensuring complete asepsis of hypodermic needles)[6] or the after-effects of a number of drugs and toxic substances, tend to be adversely affected before those with a healthy liver. In rat experiments it has been found that stress due to lack of oxygen from whatever cause in the uterus (i.e. before birth), causes degenerative changes in the liver.[7] Furthermore, the liver plays a major part in the preparation and storage of brain nutrients and, if affected by toxins, it can fail to supply the brain and nervous system with these essentials.[8]

The brain, of all our organs, seems the worst equipped to cope with deprivation. Since its need for oxygen is exacting and unceasing, it cannot make do with any substitute. When the oxygen is reduced to half the amount required, the victim rarely feels acute distress, but falls to the ground having quietly fainted. Should recovery occur, the effects of this period of severely reduced oxygen may be felt for days, or even for life, unless treatment with oxygen under pressure has been given. The cells of the central nervous system are indeed so sensitive to lack of oxygen that a rough grip or blow on the neck compressing the blood vessels to the brain can cause death very quickly. It has been estimated that the cortex suffers permanent injury if the blood supply (carrying the oxygen) is cut off for five minutes, the mid-brain for ten minutes, the medulla for fifteen to twenty minutes and the spinal cord for fifteen to thirty-five minutes, because the metabolism of these cells is very high and they cease to work when deprived of oxygen for these periods. The nerve fibres, however, work at a lower rate and will respond to stimulation after a considerable period.[9]

Those most vulnerable to a lack of oxygen caused by the combination of CO and oxygen in the blood are, in roughly descending order of magnitude: the unborn, the infant, the pregnant, those with liver or various other disabilities, and the elderly. The infant breathes more rapidly, and in proportion to its size consumes a larger quantity of air than the adult. The pregnant require oxygen for the unborn as well as for themselves. Those over-weight, or with lowered vitality or respiratory or circulatory difficulty and the elderly or aging, are more prone to react unfavourably than the healthy. Again, it has been found that any factor which speeds up respiration or circulation, such as fever, anaemia, exercise or extra activity, shortens the period before signs of the so-called CO poisoning become apparent.

An interesting sidelight on the fact that even the ultra-healthy can be affected by CO when their respiration has been increased by extra effort is provided by an incident in the Marathon Championship held at Port Elizabeth in South Africa in 1964. Disregarding, or perhaps not aware of, the precautions taken in New Zealand to protect those competing by closing the road used for the Marathon to motor traffic, and keeping official cars at a safe distance, a large number of cars closely accompanied the leaders. With four miles of the twenty-six still to go they were running strongly. Then, for no apparent reason, they began to stagger and barely managed to reach the finishing post, where they had to be given medical attention. It was considered that the fumes of CO from the accompanying cars were responsible for their distress, although these were athletic young men at the top of their form.

Differential diagnosis of CO poisoning
Dr W. F. von Oettingen, the German poisons expert, has pointed out

that a doctor may be unaware that chronic CO poisoning is the underlying cause of many chronic conditions such as some psychoses, depression, Parkinson's disease, a predisposition to bed sores, etc.[10]

In the USA in 1952 Dr Harold T. Fuerst, epidemiologist to the Department of Health of New York City, published a warning that a number of outbreaks of illness reported to his Department as food poisoning were in fact found to be CO poisoning.[11] Both of these showed nausea and vomiting, but could be differentially diagnosed by observing the following differences:

Symptoms and factors in food poisoning	Symptoms and factors in CO poisoning
Diarrhoea is the rule	Diarrhoea is rare
Headache is rare	Headache is the rule
Occurs late, resulting in vomiting, diarrhoea and dehydration	Occurs early, from weakness and blood vessel collapse
Always a pale face	Generally cyanosed (bluish) with cherry red lips, but *may* be pale faced
A common meal, and group gets ill in limited time afterwards	No common meal. Become ill simultaneously in crowded or enclosed place. Can trace to unlit or blocked gas burner, defective heater, refrigerator, leak in pipe or other source of incomplete combustion or with insufficient ventilation

Acute CO poisoning

For the average healthy adult, a rough classification of the symptoms to be expected in relation to the amount of carboxyhaemoglobin (CO present in the blood) has been stated as follows:[12]

From 1 to 10 per cent there will be no symptoms, or merely slight shortness of breath on exertion.

From 10 to 20 per cent there will be mild headache, tightness across the forehead and breathlessness on moderate exertion.

From 20 to 30 per cent there will be a throbbing headache with sensation of pressure on top of the head, irritability, emotional instability, impaired judgement and memory, and rapid fatigue.

From 30 to 40 per cent there will be severe headache, nausea and vomiting, dizziness, dimness of sight, confusion and weakness.

From 40 to 50 per cent will result in increasing confusion, staggering gait, rapid breathing and collapse on attempted exertion.

And so on until at 80 per cent there is rapid death from the cessation of breathing due to the effect on the respiratory centre in the brain.

The absorption and resulting symptoms from the inhalation of CO depend closely on: 1 The concentration of CO in the inspired air. 2 The length of time of the exposure. 3 The state of activity of the exposed person.

1 Exposure to 100 ppm for eight hours while at work will not produce symptoms in a healthy adult (but see earlier paragraph for those more vulnerable).

2 Exposure to 500 ppm for one hour may cause only slight headache and shortness of breath, with the blood carrying approximately 20 per cent of carboxyhaemoglobin. Longer exposure or greater activity raises the saturation rate to 40 to 50 per cent, causing headache, nausea, increased respiration, emotional instability, chest pains, confused impaired judgement, staggering gait, loss of sensation in the limbs and finally, if exertion is increased, fainting with lips red or blue.

3 Exposure to 1000 ppm can cause death from cessation of breathing due to the effect on the respiratory centre in the brain.

Physical examination will reveal a livid colour and a positive Romberg reaction, i.e. inability to stand upright with the feet together and, on laboratory examination, that there is increased carboxyhaemoglobin concentrated in the blood, leukocytosis and proteinuria.[13]

In acute cases not ending in coma there is mental confusion resembling drunkenness. In France a tragic case was that of the judicial execution of a woman found, apparently helpless from alcohol, by the corpses of her husband and brother. Later fatal accidents in the same house revealed that all the deaths had been due to intermittent CO fumes from a nearby lime kiln.[14]

In 1958 the *Canadian Medical Association Journal* carried an article entitled 'CO asphyxia, a common clinical entity'.[15] In the previous three years the author had personally attended thirty cases treated by Carbogen and eleven by medical attention and rest, using the spouses as a control. The cases occurred among garage workers, vehicle drivers and housewives, who made up 25 per cent of the total. The Public Health Department had surveyed local garages in the health register, and found that not enough care was taken over CO, there was inadequate ventilation, and air tests were not regularly carried out. Samples of air taken showed they were near to the maximum allowed concentration of 100 ppm. During the windy winter of 1956 there were many cases of CO poisoning in the home, mostly affecting housewives, but installing effective chimney caps cleared all the down-draughts in chimneys chiefly responsible for indoor fumes. Routine tests for carboxyhaemoglobin have since been carried out on all garage workers. Incidentally, in two cases in the home *no* leak or defects of any kind were discovered in a propane furnace or another running on oil, but the offending fumes were removed by the use of the chimney cap preventing down-draughts.

Sub-acute CO poisoning
Many conditions share the symptoms of sub-acute CO poisoning, but one clue to diagnosis is that the victim collapses on making a minor or moderate effort, due to inadequate oxygenation of the brain. This is illustrated by the case of a 47-year-old baker in the USA. After shovelling a little snow, he went up to his third floor apartment, 'sweated cold' and collapsed. He had had previous dizzy spells for which he had been given vitamin B_{12} injections. He consulted another doctor after a day in bed and he was found to be pale, not acutely distressed and with no positive findings on examination. On being questioned he said he had worked five months at his new job and *was aware of no fumes* (author's italics) but he did use an old gas cooker for heating icing sugar. He usually spent ten minutes at intervals over this stove and had noticed that some of the jets appeared defective. Two other bakers got headaches if they used it and their employer also had frequent headaches. The latter promptly had the stove repaired and the symptoms of them all abated.[16] If a percipient physician had not spotted the cause, the unsuspected danger might have had serious results for several people.

Mild CO poisoning is a known industrial hazard at gas works, but analysis of the air there is not the whole story. A laboratory attendant, reading a wet and dry bulb thermometer inserted in the main, took out the wet bulb which should have been hermetically sealed. But it was not. When he complained of head pains, he was tested in a breathing bag. It was found that the CO in this man's haemoglobin had risen from 4·7 to 12·4 per cent during the few minutes he was on the job.[17]

Chronic CO poisoning

Both before and since acute CO poisoning was accepted as a disability subject to compensation in occupational exposure, the question of whether chronic CO poisoning exists has been constantly debated. Up to 1949 the best review of the subject was that by the Danish Dr Grut, based on studies of Scandinavians driving vehicles, during some of the war years, run on producer and charcoal gas instead of petrol. Agreeing with most European writers that chronic CO poisoning does exist, he writes: 'While it is impossible to prove the existence of disease, the main characteristics of which are subjective, and present such uncharacteristic objective symptoms as CO poisoning, nevertheless, where a previously healthy individual exhibits a series of symptoms relating to CO exposure, the CO must be considered the probable cause and the disease must be treated as probably existing.'[18]

A report from Hamburg in 1960 summarized informed current medical opinion on chronic CO poisoning as follows: 'In the interest of employees and insured, whose protection is the point, it would be unjust to deny, from the clinical point of view, the existence of chronic CO poisoning whose existence is uncontested in other countries, e.g. France and Switzerland.'[19]

Although chronic CO poisoning is not scheduled as an industrial disease in Britain, the existence of a cumulative effect of CO is accepted in technical circles.[20]

In 1964, Dr Robert H. Dreisbach, in his classic book on poisoning, pointed out that although it is believed that CO does not accumulate in the body, repeated lack of oxygen from CO will cause damage to the central nervous system, with:

1 Lack of sensation in the fingers.
2 Impairment of memory.
3 Deterioration of mental ability.
4 Positive Romberg sign, i.e. swaying of the body when standing with eyes closed and the feet together.[21]

At a symposium on air pollution in 1964, a Swedish doctor reported her experiments carried out in 1955–8 on healthy persons exposed to small concentrations of CO. Her results suggested that a cumulative effect might arise from daily exposure to CO giving from 10 to 11 per cent carboxyhaemoglobin, and this was due not only to lack of oxygen but to the possibility of a block of enzymes in the respiration of tissues, and/or the accumulation of the intermediate breakdown product of foods. It was noted that there was a more persistent effect in younger subjects (from 19 to 39) whose blood vessels contracted and dilated more readily.[22]

An evaluation of the risk of chronic intoxication from the inhalation of small quantities of CO, reported in 1965 from the University of Turin's Institute of Clinical Medicine, considered that the difficulty of defining a picture of chronic CO intoxication, with its vague unspecific symptoms, justified further research into methods of diagnosis and prevention of this disability. It was concluded that such pathological states as broncho-pneumonia, addiction to smoking and anaemia aggravated the risk of intoxication.[23]

It was formerly considered that the effects of inhaling CO were entirely reversible, since they were confined to the haemoglobin, but there is now evidence that this is not so. Experimental work with rabbits has shown that after a certain period CO collects and accumulates in the plasma. After the CO ceased to be given, there was a lowering of the CO in the red blood cells, but a quantity remained in the plasma for a long period. They found the CO linked with the extra haemoglobin iron which may explain why in chronic poisoning there is not a significant increase in carboxyhaemoglobin. It had already been shown that in chronic CO poisoning with small concentrations of CO, the oxygen consumption in the tissues was clearly lowered. Symptoms might include disturbance of balance, smell, hearing and vision, and might progress even after the cessation of exposure to CO.[24]

Where the worker in France is known to be at risk in his occupation (though probably inhaling less CO than a housewife exposed to unvented or malfunctioning sources of CO) it has been recommended that every case of poisoning, however light, should be reported as a works accident, and supervised by the works doctor, who should follow the course of the later effects and protect the rights of the victim. A typical case where this was not done and which had a very serious outcome was that of a patient never off work or reporting sick, though he had suffered repeated slight sub-acute symptoms, who was sent to a neuro-psychologist. He diagnosed Parkinson's disease, attributable to an acute poisoning incident followed by chronic poisoning, showing insignificant amounts of CO in his blood, which is a characteristic of chronic CO intoxication. Unfortunately, a very full programme of restorative measures had little effect on the disability, which was considered progressive.[25]

Effects on performance
A series of experiments with eighteen young adults revealed that even low concentrations of CO impair performance, though no discomfort is felt and the subject cannot reliably judge whether any CO is present. Each was tested in an enclosed booth with CO added in concentrations of 0, 50, 100, 175 and 250 ppm. Over four-hour periods each person was given 600 tests, with rest breaks. With only 50 ppm there were deteriorations in performance after ninety minutes, to the surprise of the researchers. None felt discomfort or was aware that CO was present.[26]

Research has been undertaken, under the direction of Dr Ewan Cameron of the Albany Hospital of the US Veterans' Administration, on individuals of all ages who suffer mental deficits because of CO poisoning; it is intended to help these people with magnesium pemoline, a new memory drug.[27]

It is to be hoped that their researches may lead to the lowering of the MAC (maximum allowable concentration)* of 100 ppm for atmospheric pollution in work places in Britain and the USA to the more realistic figure of 20 ppm, with the eventual target of 16 ppm now current in the USSR.

It is possible, with the aid of electrical techniques, to detect happenings in the cortex, that part of the brain connected with the mind. This demonstrates that it is more sensitive to deficiency of oxygen than the rest of the brain. A shortage here can lead to disturbances of thought and even derangement of ideas. A distinct decrease in the aptitude for mathematics has been frequently observed at high altitudes. This suggests the possibility that part of a similar lack of aptitude in the young might be relieved if oxygen shortages due to CO in the atmosphere of home and school buildings were to be thoroughly investigated and corrected. Two most important masses of nerve cells in the grey matter of the brain are concerned with the expression of the emotions, and react so sensitively to the quality of the surrounding fluids that any reduction in their supply of oxygen can lead to anything from a lack of mental activity to unconsciousness. The adjacent sleep centre can also be so disturbed

* Called MPC in Britain—maximum permissible concentration.

by an oxygen shortage as to upset the ability to sleep naturally, which no amount of sleeping pills can be expected to put right. In fact, as Professor Ashley Montagu has pointed out, 'The physiological nature of the reactivity of the nervous system at any given time can be altered by the action of substances circulating in the blood such as toxins and gases.'[28]

Other domestic sources of CO and other fumes
Undoubtedly wood was the first fuel of man and it is still employed where other fuels are dear and scarce. Since it invariably produces CO, it should never be burned without an outlet. A case reported from Uruguay is a warning of the severity of the penalty paid for neglecting this precaution. A healthy 24-year-old workman lit a wood stove in an unventilated bedroom. Nine hours later he was found unconscious, having fallen in a corner of the room. He remained in a coma for five days, developed a serious ulcer on the back and presented the appearance of a disease of the central nervous system known as Parkinson's or paralysis agitans.[29]

The universal use of charcoal in the Middle Ages is said to have caused many deaths in the poorly ventilated though draughty dwellings. In Spain today, where really cold days are fortunately few, the use of charcoal persists in braziers and not only in the humbler and remoter districts. Charcoal is smokeless, but gives off fumes of CO while glowing, so can be dangerous when lighted—or extinguished. It is popularly supposed that it is not used indoors until all the CO has been burnt out, and removed from any room that is to be slept in. Anyone familiar with the Spanish horror of night air coming in through an open window will heave a sigh of relief at this information. In France, cooks using charcoal for cooking and launderers using charcoal irons have suffered anaemia from continued absorption of CO, a familiar disability to French physicians. There appears to be no such occurrences in Britain, where charcoal is no longer used except for the modern barbecue, luckily an outdoor usage. However, in Persia, the custom of sitting round the 'Corsi' still claims its child victims. There is a low round table with a brazier underneath in the centre, the whole structure being covered with a thick quilt and then a tablecloth. Families and their guests sit round on the floor with their legs extended towards the centre and tuck the edge of the tablecloth under their chins. When children in play crawl under the quilt, as they frequently do, they are suffocated by fumes since the porosity of charcoal makes it produce more CO than any other solid fuel.[30]

For many years it has been traditional among miners to keep coal fires burning day and night, as they get a concession of about eight tons of coal a year. This domestic smoke blows down to breathing level, and must be held responsible for the fact that more cases of bronchitis occur in mining areas than anywhere else in Britain, where the total death rate from this disease is 32,000 yearly or nearly a hundred a day. Today miners in smokeless zones are given an annual grant enabling them to buy smokeless fuel. Although this has some effect on health and cleanliness it is not enough, for, as we have seen, these fuels still produce fumes which are harmful.

Dangers and disabilities caused by gas
For ten years Dr Theron Randolph in the USA has thoroughly studied and treated the clinical effects of domestic air pollution and gas in particular. He has found that whether or not a person is aware of the impingement on health by chemical air pollution depends on the degree of susceptibility and the frequency of exposure. He warns that slight leaks may occur from every pilot and other automatic device on a gas appliance which can go undetected by an inspector; that down draughts through an unused fireplace from a double chimney carrying both fire and furnace flues may foul the adjacent room, though this can be obviated by keeping a fire going when the adjacent flue is used in a wind; that furnaces should always be outside the living quarters, in a room entered only from outside; that gas refrigerators in small kitchens are major causes of trouble; and that gas cookers are so guilty that he has removed them in 500 cases, the expense being justified in the eyes of the patient by the clinical improvement. The major indictment of his report refers to fuel-oil or gas space heaters and gas wall heaters and cookers without a vent.[31] His conclusions have been confirmed by responsible investigators in many European countries.

This illuminating and extensive report is published in *Annals of Allergy*. The definition of allergy given by the *Oxford English Diction-ary* is: 'A condition of unusual or exaggerated susceptibility to a substance which is harmless in similar amounts for the majority of members of the same species.' Yet the common factor in all the conditions affecting the health of Dr Randolph's patients was *chemical pollutants*, to which every warm-blooded animal reacts unfavourably in some degree. His findings therefore have significance for us all.

It is easy to understand the popularity of gas with cooks unaware of its dangers if not correctly installed and maintained. To quote an expert on heating and ventilation: 'Coal gas for cooking is economical, as it can be turned off when not wanted and turned on again at once. *Of course it ought not to be left unprovided with a chimney.*'[32] (Author's italics.) The chimney should also have a down-draught prevention cap, as down-draughts often extinguish pilot lights. It is very seldom that this safety clause about providing a chimney is observed. It should be clearly understood that the burning of gas in any household appliance not fitted with a vent or flue leads to pollution of the household air. This is especially true in winter when, with most windows closed, noxious fumes trapped within the walls cannot diffuse and disperse as they can out of doors.

There are many varieties of gas in common use. Town gas is a mixture of methane, CO and traces of hydrogen sulphide and naphthalene. Its CO content makes it lighter than air and very toxic, but it does not form pockets. It burns to CO_2, water, SO_2 and sooty stuff making a scale on cooking utensils, and CO when incompletely burned. Calor and Botogas are propane and butane extracted from the waste gas of oil refineries. They are not toxic but asphyxiating, since they are *heavier* than air and displace this in the lower parts of confined spaces, which makes them dangerous for boats, caravans and tents, though they burn very cleanly, forming little but CO_2 and water if they have an adequate air supply.

A couple, accidentally asphyxiated in a motor vessel at sea off Plymouth in 1967, had died from the CO fumes from their calor gas cooker. This seems to underline the commonsense practice in Spain (where Botogas is in very common use in the kitchens) of placing a chimney directly over every cooker, although constant ventilation through open doorways and windows may be taken for granted in such a hot climate.

On 21 December 1965 Mr Fred Lee, Minister of Power, said in the House of Commons that Great Britain should be able to receive at least fifty million cubic feet daily from the natural gas deposits in the North Sea. This consists mainly of methane, which has twice the heating value of coal gas. It is widely claimed and believed that *methane* contains no carbon monoxide, and this of course is quite true. It is often diluted, however, with carbon monoxide to enable it to be used in old-fashioned burners, and, like all combustible materials, it can also produce CO by incomplete combustion and the reduction of CO_2 in its products. An article in the *New Scientist* (12 September 1963) gave the following important information:

'By 1968 Regional Gas Boards expect to reduce the CO content of domestic gas to 5 per cent, a level which they claim is safe. Though this is not the opinion of experts. As long as gas was obtained entirely from the combustion of coal as it was in its early years, it only contained from 5 to 10 per cent CO. Later, the mixture of water and producer gas made from coke by two different methods raised this figure to about 20 per cent. Since the inhalation of gas with this high percentage is rapidly fatal, there were an increasing number of accidental deaths from this cause, which has prompted the Gas Boards to reduce the percentage by mixing gas from oil with natural gas from the Sahara. They still only aim at 5 per cent, so that a would-be suicide can still use a gas oven—only it will take longer to die—though it will undoubtedly reduce the number of accidental deaths from leaking pipes or defective domestic appliances.'

No gas can really be considered safe unless the CO and SO_2 produced in use is removed by venting to below the maximum permissible concentration (MPC) allowed by British law in any place where men and women are employed for eight hours daily. As far as the housewife is concerned, she is at liberty to inhale just as much of this deleterious pollutant as her domestic appliances can and do supply throughout the far longer hours she works in her home.

Come for a tour of some such home and you will understand what is involved. Here is a kitchen where a mid-day meal for the family is being prepared and will soon be served. It is not very large, but it is a cold, wet day so the ground floor window, which has been closed all night, is hardly open at all. A large very up-to-date gas cooker stands against the inner wall. There are three steaming saucepans on all but one of the rings that lie on each side of a central line where a pilot jet burns day and night. The cooking jets have been turned to low since the contents of the saucepans reached boiling point about half an hour ago. A joint is roasting and an apple pie baking in the oven which is also turned fairly low. Quite a large amount of gas is obviously burning. Where, we ask, is the overhead chimney, canopy or funnelling vent necessary to carry off the considerable volume of

CO that must be given off by so much simultaneous combustion of carbon with oxygen? There is none.

Over the double sink hangs a medium size geyser providing constant hot water, with the flame of its pilot jet burning night and day. Since this is a very particular housewife, who always washes socks and cardigans rather than trust them to her washing machine, and clears up her dirty utensils as she goes along, this water heater has been in fairly constant use ever since she washed up the breakfast dishes. Again we note that there is no sign of any vent to carry away the fumes which are inevitably confined in this not very large enclosed space.

No one in his senses installs a range or a coal-burning grate without a chimney behind it to carry off the smoke containing the CO that can maim or even kill. The many generations of gas cookers which displaced kitchen ranges inherited a chimney, but modern gas cookers do not. Even geysers in bathrooms are not uncommon causes of fatalities although they are never to be found without a venting chimney. This is because they are frequently not secured against accidental blockage, such as birds' nests, or they may lack a down-draught preventing cap. Why are not all gas water heaters as installed in kitchens supplied with these essential devices? Enquiry at a local gas office elicits the complacent but surely question-begging reply that, as they are only burning for short periods, such a vent is not deemed necessary. This may be the official view of companies supplying the appliance, but it does not tally with two facts. A water heater over a kitchen sink may frequently be in use for a series of not-so-short periods which amount to a considerable time. In the opinion of such noteworthy experts as the biological chemist Donald E. Carr: 'All burners should have a flue to channel the burnt gas out of the house,' though, as he comments, and we can confirm from a great deal of personal observation, 'this is far from universal or even common practice the world over'.[33] As he explains, it is important to realize that when a multi-jet burner is turned low, the gas may burn completely to water and safe carbon dioxide only in a *percentage* of the orifices. The holes which are partly plugged may emit gas, which at lower-than-flame temperature produce CO and other fumes. How often, too, does milk or a pan of potatoes boil over and extinguish some of the flame, leaving some of the orifices partly plugged up when the flame is turned down to prevent it boiling over again?

Unvented panel heaters and radiant heaters are on sale in every gas showroom, and are constantly to be found in the halls of new houses and on the walls of restaurants, although it is specifically laid down by the British Standards Institution that such appliances should have 'the products of combustion discharged into a chimney or flue', and that 'where an appliance requiring a flue is to be fitted in a room which is not already provided with a flue, a *permanent flue of an adequate area not normally less than 20 square inches should be installed*'.[34] (Author's italics.) Why is this so blatantly disregarded? Customers may not sit long over a meal, but employees should not be exposed to such fumes throughout their working day.*

Since July 1966 there has been a spectacular leap in sales of gas heaters, cookers and central heating appliances, especially the latter, which totalled 138,900 in 1967–8, a rise of 14 per cent on the previous year. There is room for much more than complacency over these figures.

The Ronan Point disaster in London in 1968 drew public attention to the serious results of gas explosions in tall blocks of 'system built' flats, and now, by government order, electrical appliances are to replace gas in similarly constructed buildings, and new building regulations now apply.

The French Government, after two years of discussion on the safety or otherwise of gas for cooking and refrigeration in high buildings, had already vetoed its use in such places as being too dangerous. As few French women cook with gas this has not caused the complaints raised in England where 70 per cent of women do, clinging to it with a fanatical obstinacy which ignores its drawbacks and dangers. For the British Government to follow the French lead, overriding uninformed outcries, would be a praiseworthy measure, removing a number of gas appliances potentially menacing not only the health of many more unsuspected victims of fumes from this source, but the lives of hundreds. Here are figures applying to accidental deaths in England and Wales, supplied by the Royal Society for the Prevention of Accidents, for 1963 and 1966 (the last

* The Shops and Railway Premises Act 1963 stipulates that 'no method of securing and maintaining a reasonable temperature (in which persons are employed to work otherwise than for short periods) shall be used which results in the escape into the air of any fumes (including gas and vapour) of such a character as to be likely to be injurious or offensive to persons working therein'. But unlike factories and workshops, etc., these premises have no inspectors to ensure this statutory protection.

period for which full details are available) and the total of accidental gas deaths in 1967:

	1963	1966	1967
Total domestic accidental deaths	8024	1740	not available
Deaths from all gases and vapours	1329	866	785
Deaths from household gas	1236	790	711

The prevention of tragedies probably due to gas central heating or pockets of cold air blocking flue outlets and causing fumes in the hot air ducts should also receive attention from experts. One such case of the former occurred in a newly built open-plan suburban house on Christmas Day 1966, where two guests and a dog died after eating their Christmas dinner and the two other diners were taken to hospital seriously ill from the same cause.

In another incident nearly two years later on a new housing estate, three people and two canaries were found dead from asphyxiation. According to the New Town manager, investigation revealed no fault in the gas central heating. In fact, there appears to have been an improper flue, as there is a requirement that 'flame out' valves must be installed in case of down-draughts, even if there is a down-draught cap on the vent. The seven families of the other flats with this same, supposedly foolproof, system were warned not to shut all their windows so as to ensure adequate ventilation!—hardly a safe or pleasant solution. This is a situation which deserves the enquiry it has not yet received in order to prevent not only the occurrence of more deaths, but those less tragic cases of disabilities attributable to the same cause.

In 1942, after prolonged and careful study, a USA physician reported that 150 patients, whose illness could be definitely traced to the effects of *natural* gas used in appliances *which were not vented*, showed that 'CO from improper combustion of natural gas, chiefly through defective heating appliances, is often responsible for chronic states of ill-health, and constitutes a problem which needs further study and investigation'.[35]

More than one coroner has warned that the increasingly popular use of double glazing, fitted carpets, and other draught excluders can dangerously affect the return air flow of gas-fired warm air central heating. Investigations following four deaths from CO poisoning in 1968 showed that forty-five minutes after such a heating system had been turned on, the CO content built up in the living-room to a lethal figure because of the draught exclusion measures previously taken.

In France in 1950, Dr Vallaud warned that, owing to the existence in old houses of communicating chimneys (which ought to be prohibited), people might be poisoned by gases liberated by the heating or cooking appliances of other inhabitants of the house, and referred to a hundred cases of chronic CO poisoning recorded in forty-six reports which were published in 1943. In thirty-nine of these cases there were fissures in chimney casings, and nine of the other cases were due to lighting gas.[36]

Of course, there are British Standards Institution Codes of Practice dealing with the installation of all gas appliances, but BSI has no power to compel compliance. These codes state categorically that flueless appliances may be installed only where there is 'adequate ventilation'. This seems to leave the way wide open to individual interpretations of what is adequate, which may be much less than desirable. In giving general guidance, however, it is clearly stated that a flue must be fitted where a room is small, or in a confined space with poor ventilation, or where usage is likely to be heavy. Furthermore, hoods and canopies to collect products of combustion steam, etc., and remove them *via a flue* are recommended since they also function as down-draught diverters and assist general ventilation.[37] But, of course, those purchasing second-hand cookers, refrigerators or heaters generally have no idea of the possible dangers of ignorance in fitting these appliances, and have probably never heard of BSI, much less of these Codes of Practice.

Gas in everyday life in the USSR
The indifferent and permissive official attitude in this country where domestic pollution by gas is concerned can be contrasted with that in the USSR in recent years. For example, a paper was published in 1962 concerning Uzbekistan where, in 1957, gas was supplied to only 4801 flats, but an estimated 400,000 people would be supplied in 1965. This specified that a gas stove must not be used with the 'fortochka' (the small one-paned window present in most Russian rooms) *closed, even if there is a ventilation channel*, for 'without access of fresh air to the kitchen, the concentration of CO may rise to an unacceptable amount'. So the 'fortochka' must be open day and night. It is stressed that the use of large, flat utensils limits the access

of air and increases the undesirable products of combustion. Pointing out that the general change over to natural gas is the most effective way of reducing the CO content of air to the permitted level, it is emphasized that though gas stoves in kitchens only give out small amounts of CO, this often exceeds the permitted domestic amount of 16 ppm. The industrial limit is 24 ppm in the USSR. Figures from the publication quoted above are given showing that investigations in Moscow had found concentrations of 256 ppm to 528 ppm, in Lvov of 260 ppm to 464 ppm and in Leningrad of 56 ppm. It is concluded that if the products of combustion are carried off through a 'smoke-vent', pollution of the kitchen air with CO can be eliminated completely, and plans for such a stove have been produced.[38]

Paraffin cookers and heaters
Paraffin is a distillate oil with a low sulphur content. Its worst product in burning is CO which is produced either by insufficient draught, hot soot or hot metal parts. In this country it is coloured for home use and smells slightly, probably producing oxides of nitrogen and sulphur. Cookers using paraffin, if not burning completely or not kept scrupulously clean, will always emit noxious fumes, yet they are *never* given a flue or vent. In the past, heaters have been notoriously dangerous sources of fire. They now have a built-in safety device which automatically puts out the burner flame if the heater is over-turned, lifted or tilted more than fifteen degrees from the vertical.[39] But the Oil Heater Regulations 1963 (as amended 1966) only deal with fire prevention, and fatalities still occur from the fumes emitted.

In a case reported on Boxing Day 1965, a paraffin-type heater was found alight beside the dead bodies of five members of a family sitting in a van. In another case, a husband awoke to find his infant son dead in a cot and his wife unconscious, because of an oil heater he had lighted before going to bed. His wife died later in hospital, but he and two small children recovered. The coroner remarked that incomplete combustion from the heater could have produced a poisonous atmosphere in the room, and death from CO fumes was confirmed by a pathologist. It is possible for any oil heater to burn with incomplete combustion and give off these dangerous fumes, but they are never given a suitably placed vent. It has been estimated that in every house in multiple occupation, at least one portable oil heater is in use which does not comply with the legal standards of safety laid down. This is bad enough from the fire risk involved, but perhaps equally disturbing because of the noxious fumes produced.

The primus stove so popular with campers and caravanners also gives off CO whenever it is burning, and ten times more so when in use for cooking. Therefore it should only be used out of doors and never in small enclosed spaces, especially not in tents in cold, still conditions when the permeability of the walls is reduced and the CO cannot escape.

Acts of Parliament deal more or less effectively with the dangers of pollution in public places. To whom can we look for a solution to the problems of domestic pollution outlined in this chapter? Surely these must be given our own urgent individual attention before any sort of regulating legislation can be invoked.

REFERENCES

1 MARANZANA, P. *et al. Rassegna de Medicina Indust.*, Vol. 33, 3–4 (1964)
2 SMITH, ALAN R. *Air Pollution Monograph No. 28* (Society of Chemical Industry, 1965)
3 BIERSTREKER, K. *et al* 'Indoor Air Pollution in Rotterdam', *Int. Jour. Air Pollution* (Pergamon Press, 1965)
4 SPEIZER, F. E. *et al. Arch. Environ. Health*, 12, No. 6 (June 1966)
5 SHERLOCK, SHEILA. *The Liver in Circulatory Diseases* (Philadelphia, 1956)
6 THE STERILISATION, USE AND CARE OF SYRINGES, MRC memo No. 41 (HMSO, 1962)
7 GRUENWALD, P. *Am. Jour. Clin. Path.*, Dreisbach, 19, 861, (1949)
8 CAMPBELL, D. G. *Jour. Digest. Disturb.*, Vol. 1, 342 (August 1956)
9 DREISBACH, ROBERT H. *Handbook of Poisoning*, 4th Edition (Lange Medical Publications, 1963)
10 SCHENK, GUSTAV. *The Book of Poisons* (Weidenfeld & Nicolson, 1956)
11 *Science Newsletter* (20 July 1952)
12 DREISBACH, ROBERT H. *Handbook of Poisoning*, 4th Edition (Large Medical Publications, 1963)
13 *Ibid.*
14 RAYMOND, V., VALLAUD, A. *Leçons de Toxicologie*, Vol. III (Hermann et Cie, Paris, 1943)
15 KATZ, M. *Can. Med. Ass. Jour.*, Vol. 78 (1 February 1958)
16 BELL, MILTON A. *Arch. of Environ. Health*, Vol. 3. (November 1961)
17 MINCHIN, L. T. *Coke and Gas*, 16, 425 (1954)
18 GRUT, A. *Chronic CO Poisoning* (Munksgaard, Copenhagen, 1949)
19 PETRY, H. *Arch. für Gewerbe p.u. Gewerbehyg 18*, 22–36 (Hamburg, 1960)
20 HILLS, J. B. G., B.SC. Personal Communication
21 DREISBACH, ROBERT H. *Handbook of Poisoning*, 4th Edition (Lange Medical Publications, 1963)
22 VON POST-LINGIN, MARIE LOUISE. *Proc. of Roy. Soc. of Med.*, Vol. 57, No. 10 (October 1964)
23 PERELLI, G. *et al. Minerva Medica*, 56, Med. de Lavoro (13 October 1965)

24   PECORA, I. *et al. Fol. Med.*, Vol. 70 (1957)
25   BREUIL, M. *Arch. des Ma. Prof. du Tr. et de S. Soc.*, 144 (March 1962)
26   BEARD, R. R. *et al. Am. J. Pub. Health.*, Vol. 57, No. 11 (November 1967)
27   EUROPEAN CONFERENCE ON AIR POLLUTION (1964)
28   MONTAGU, ASHLEY. *The Direction of Human Development* (Charles C. Thomas, Illinois, 1957)
29   BERNARDINO, RODRIGUES *et al. Ann. de la Facul. de Med.*, Univ. of Montevideo, 46 (1961)
30   HILLS, J. B. G., B.SC. Personal Communication
31   RANDOLPH, THERON. *Anns. of Allergy* (19 June 1961)
32   BEDFORD, THOMAS. *Basic Principles of Ventilation and Heating* (H. K. Lewis, 1964)
33   CARR, DONALD. *The Breath of Life* (Gollancz, 1965)
34   BRITISH STANDARDS INSTITUTION Codes of Practice CP 332 (1963); CP 306 (August 1965)
35   BECK, HARVEY. *New Orleans Med. & Surg. Jour.* Vol. 94 (8 February 1942)
36   RAYMOND, V., VALLAUD, A. *CO and Chronic CO Poisoning* (Paris, 1950)
37   BRITISH STANDARDS INSTITUTION Codes of Practice CP 331, 104, 302 (1963)
38   SMOLYASK, M. *Med. Zn. Uzbek U.S.S.R.*, 6, 13, (6 January 1962)
39   Comment 'On preventing sale of unsafe oil heaters', *Municipal Engineering* (2 August 1968)

2

Clearing the Air

'The cure for this ill is not to sit still.'
                                        RUDYARD KIPLING

In the sixteenth century a deputation of women went to
see Queen Elizabeth I about 'the filthy danger in the use of coal'.
They did not suceed in their aim of putting an end to the dirt or
danger, either publicly or privately. In the reign of Queen Elizabeth
II we need not be deterred by their failure but rather inspired by their
example.

After centuries of existence as ciphers, at least nominally, women
have succeeded in breaking the barriers of custom to swarm into
polling booths, penetrate Parliament, sit in the Cabinet and throng
a thousand of the ancient preserves of man. Starting out as pioneers,
they have in a few decades turned unprecedented tasks into com-
monplaces. There remains a common task facing housewives today.
Individually and banded together they must attack and overcome
the menace of pollution in the home.

There seems little place today, if ever, for witchcraft and occult
groups, but their decision in 1969 to ban the use at their meetings of
all fuels which emit noxious fumes, 'in the interests of physical and
spiritual health', presents an instance and example of enlightenment
coming from a dark place. How do we set about banning, for the
same reason, all noxious fumes in our homes?

Measures against combustion fumes
The first step is to become aware of the presence of these invisible
moths that nibble at the wholesome fabric of domestic air. Here,
noses are not enough. It has been the custom for coal miners to
carry canaries as indicators of the presence of carbon monoxide
fumes. When these reach danger level the canary usually falls off its
perch and the miner, although he has felt no symptoms, knows he
must get out or go under. But it has been found unwise to rely

entirely on the canaries' reaction and a variety of detection devices have been tested. None of these has proved dependable, since they are affected significantly by whether they are used in still or moving air and they are put out of action by humidity. In kitchens and moving vehicles the chemicals used rapidly absorb moisture and are rendered not only useless but deceptive.[1]

Since it has been made clear that the use of any appliance for cooking or heating employing any fuel except electricity can and does produce noxious fumes, these must be assumed to be present in smaller or greater degree (even if wholly undetected) wherever special venting has not been provided. For perfect safety to health, these fumes must be removed.

Obviously, the surest way to achieve this is to change over to electric appliances. This is an expensive step, but has been considered well worthwhile by those advised to do so by their physician. But how many physicians are aware that noxious fumes may underlie many disabling conditions of health? For those households unwilling to incur this expense, there are other measures which should prove effective.

Removal by better combustion and by cowls
Practical hints on coal usage by an engineering consultant are:
- a Fire should be fitted to the size of the room. Measure the area say 15 ft by 12 ft in square feet. This gives 180 sq. ft. Then divide by 9. This is 20 sq. ft. Expressed in square inches this gives the size of the grate required to warm the room adequately, i.e. 20 square inches a grate about 7 in. by 3 in. A large grate should be reduced by fire bricks to the correct size.
- b Never let the fire fall to a dull red glow before adding fresh fuel. Add a little at a time while it is still bright and clear and HOT. The high temperature (about 900°F) ignites the gases as they are liberated. Dumping a shovelful on a fire at a low temperature *makes noxious fumes emerge*, which choke you, create soot up the chimney and waste coal. So feed little and often to keep the fire bright and clean.[2]

Fitting an adequate cowl can cure down-draught causing fumes in the room, but in the case of a low bungalow chimney this may mean directing the outpoured smoke into your own or a neighbour's windows or garden.

Makers' instructions for fuelling and refuelling with solid fuel and oil should be carefully followed. Again, cowls may be necessary to convert down-draughts into up-draughts in the chimney, but in spite of this, unfavourable winds have been known to divert the fumes through the upper floor windows.

If portable oil heaters cannot be dispensed with, they should be kept spotlessly clean, the wicks well trimmed and any room in which they are burning well ventilated at all times.

Removal by venting and good maintenance
In the case of gas appliances, the most important measure is to install appropriate venting immediately overhead to the outside air, as considered essential by ventilation experts and the British Standards Institution. Furthermore, any housewife using gas for cooking, hot water and central heating should recall a coroner's warning that adding draught excluders and fitted carpets to such a home may spell fatality if down-draughts occur. Referring to inducement reductions offered to housewives using gas only, for all purposes including central heating, the Industrial Editor of the *Sunday Times* (22 December 1968) had this to say: 'If in addition she falls for the fashion of double glazing, there is going to be *death to pay for it.*' Of course, all gas appliances should be frequently and regularly tested to ensure that all orifices are kept clean and that blockages and wear have not rendered them dangerous.

Unfortunately, under the Gas Act 1948, gas boards have no right to condemn any installation by private firms, nor to withhold supplies of gas. Nor do they inspect systems installed by approved private contractors. They should be called in consultation in such cases. Following deaths from carbon monoxide arising from faults in a gas-fired warm air system in 1967, a coroner in Sutherland called for legislation giving gas boards the power to make faulty gas installations safe, or to remove them. This advice has apparently been disregarded.

Financial assistance is available under the Clean Air Act for those facing unavoidable expenditure in the conversion of their appliances in smoke control areas. Why should not users of gas appliances, not previously provided with proper vents, be allowed similar financial assistance in fitting such vents? In addition, why has no one invented a cheap electric poker for completely safe use as an ignition instrument?

Installation of electric central heating
Where electric radiators are installed in the chimney-breast in any room of a house having an adjoining chimney where coal or solid fuels are burned, there is serious danger that air pollution will follow, yet be wholly unsuspected and undetected although causing respiratory and other trouble. Fumes can pour through the interstices in the brick construction between the two flues caused by the corrosive action on the mortar of the sulphur dioxide in the smoke of burning fires. In all such cases, the respective flues should be properly relined.

In former times the inside of a flue in a chimney stack was 'parged' with a mixture of lime mortar and cow dung which formed an impervious layer by chemical reaction. This prevented leakage between adjacent flues or through the stack into other rooms. The practice was abandoned about the turn of the century because, it is said, bricklayers objected to handling the mixture. The modern practice is to use a coarse undercoat plaster which is more porous than the bricks. Furthermore, it is usual nowadays for large heating appliances to be connected to the same porous flue that served an old-fashioned grate, and far more leakage results from the increased flow of combustion products. Some makers of central heating boilers recommend asbestos linings that can be pushed up the existing flue in sections to guard against this, but it seems they are often omitted. Better builders fit lined flues in new houses built for central heating, but in all old houses this is a matter which must receive attention, since omission to do so may have dangerous consequences for the occupants.[3]

'Air improvers'
There are many variations on the theme of hood, canopy, filter, air purifier and so on on the modern market, which claim to remove fumes, dust, bacteria, smoke, etc. These claims should be looked at with a wary eye and some important facts should be borne in mind before deciding to spend money on any of these magical inventions. These facts can be summarized as follows:

   a Those dispensing fragrant essential oils act as deodorants, banishing smells by replacing unpleasant ones by pleasant. Provided they contain no hydrocarbons, these are not deleterious. They can do nothing, however, to alter the composition of the air.

b Those operating through a filter of activated carbon can absorb all the toxic and inert gases, with the important *exception* of carbon monoxide.

c Those circulating moisture into air which has been over-dried by central heating have value as humidifiers. They can hardly justify any claim to dispel stuffiness on hot summer days in the British climate, since such days are usually high in humidity.

d Fan units vary in efficiency, but perform a useful function in moving air, so assisting the natural cooling of the body, but this movement is likely to be ineffective in very humid conditions.

e Those producing ozone have a nasty habit of emitting oxides of nitrogen, which may react with all sorts of hydrocarbons, proprietary polishes and detergents to produce eye irritants. These irritants include ozone itself, a notorious ingredient in the Los Angeles 'smog', where it arises from the action of sunlight on nitrous oxides from car exhausts.[4]

Ozone not so healthy

Ozone is frequently regarded as a symbol of fresh air, but in fact the so-called 'smell of ozone' on a beach is that of iodine released by decaying seaweed.[5] It is popularly believed to be beneficial to man but in fact, it can be very toxic. The addition of one atom too many of life's guardian angel oxygen (O_2) changes it to ozone (O_3) which can be an enemy to life. A question of position is involved. In their proper place in the lifeless atmosphere some 80,000 feet up, ozone atoms hover like kindly bird wings to protect the earth from the sun and to keep its temperature stable. Let them come down to the level of the air we breathe and they begin to resemble vultures.

In 1960, Professor C. A. Mills reported that there were some 400 deaths a year from respiratory and cardiac disease in Los Angeles 'smogs' when the level of ozone rose about 0·1 ppm.[6] Workers at the University of Groningen, Holland, in 1964 produced evidence that, in man and in experimental animals, breathing air containing ozone at concentrations of 0·2 ppm to 0·25 ppm causes effects on cells similar to the damage caused by radiation.[7]

In America, H. E. Stokinger and his co-workers, carrying out brilliant extensive and methodical investigations of ozone toxicity, have stated that there has been a rise in the prevalence of ozone as an air pollutant owing to its presence in Los Angeles 'smog'; in un-pressurized aircraft cabins at altitudes of over 30,000 feet; in inert gas shielded arc-welding and in a wave of ozone-producing devices for air purification. Reviewing the years 1954 to 1964 in this field, they reported that while useful in destroying moulds and bacteria which spoil cheese, this usefulness *did not apply* to the addition of ozone to the ventilation of inhabited premises for air sterilization.[8]

Ozone not so effective

Many years ago it was found that at 0·015 ppm, but not below that level, ozone reduced body odour by *masking* it.[9] According to an eminent modern ventilation expert, 'ozone is NOT a practicable germicide for use in ventilation'. It can only inactivate bacteria when there are simple aerosol particles in 60 to 90% relative humidity, and in a humid room only a trace of its given output is obtained, but on a dry day this may become undesirably high.[10]

As for the effect of ozone as a domestic 'air improver', the lecturer at a conference arranged by the Medical Information Service in Munich in 1962 summed up the evidence as follows: 'The effect of ozone is therefore a psychological trick achieved by a partial anaesthesia of the mucous membrane of the nose. Furthermore, the trick has the disadvantage that ozone belongs to those gases which do not refresh man but tire him.'[11]

Fatalities and near-fatalities from gas fumes

In 1965 there were 806 accidental deaths from household gas in England and Wales (but only fifty-seven from electricity).[12] Every year old people, those with an inadequate sense of smell, children, heavy sleepers and others are the victims of fumes from gas appliances. Many of these cases, with respiration so badly affected that they were formerly not expected to revive, can now be resuscitated through transference to an atmosphere of oxygen under pressure. The first unit of this kind was built at the Western Infirmary, Glasgow, where it was shown that dogs gassed with carbon monoxide could be saved in this way. The victim and the resuscitating team are placed in a large cylinder in which the air is compressed to two atmospheres. While the team breathe ordinary air, the patient inhales pure oxygen under pressure from a cylinder. The effect is to raise the oxygen content of the blood so high that it drives out the toxic carbon monoxide in about forty minutes, about six times more quickly than if the patient were breathing ordinary air. The effects on heart and brain have been found eminently satisfactory in wiping out the mental disturbances so common after this form of poisoning, and in showing normal electrocardiograms within half an hour of receiving the pressurized oxygen. Of course, this form of treatment is entirely a matter for experts, but first aid is invaluable in all cases of such poisoning.

Everyone using gas in any form, whether properly vented or not, or for that matter any other kind of combustion, should be prepared to deal efficiently with accidental asphyxia where the patient will be unconscious. This may occur in a number of ways, but the result is the same. Death is imminent. What is to be done and by whom?

The first thing to remember is that it is up to the person *on the spot*. Speed of action is absolutely essential in order to save the life. Do not run to phone the doctor. Do not leave the asphyxiated person. There is grave danger of damage to the brain and other vital organs, even though life be saved, if the asphyxiated state is allowed to continue. In fact, the brain cannot take more than eight minutes of oxygen deprivation without permanent harm being inflicted.

You must act immediately yourself. You must know clearly the steps to take, and take them at once. The ambulance should be called later. Many people have died on the way to hospital who might have been saved by anyone on the spot who could carry out the well-tried method of artificial respiration which is called mouth-to-mouth or the kiss of life. Keep quite calm and proceed as follows:

1 Remove the patient from the source of danger at once. If this is not possible, turn off any leaking tap and break the windows— a shoe heel held firmly in the hand will do it.
2 Undo or cut off all tight clothing such as collar and tie, or bra, girdle, etc., and then open the front of the clothing.
3 Place the patient on the back, removing dentures if worn.
4 Put the thumb and forefinger into the mouth, grasp and pull the tongue forward if it has fallen back.
5 Kneel on either side of the patient facing the head and pressing one hand up between the shoulder-blades raise so that the head is extended with the chin uppermost. Put a handkerchief over the patient's mouth.
6 Now take a deep breath, and apply your mouth to the mouth of the patient, closing an adult's nose with the fingers of one hand, or a child's by covering nose as well as mouth with your own mouth. Blow as hard as you can. Take another breath then

blow again. Do this about ten times a minute. Keep steadily on until the chest begins to rise.

7 Remove your mouth as the chest rises and the patient will breathe out.
8 Repeat the breathing into the mouth. As soon as the chest rises again remove your mouth again and let the patient breathe out.
9 Continue this procedure until the patient is able to breathe freely without your aid.

Taking it confidently and calmly you should be able to continue for a long time until professional help can be summoned.

In cases of milder poisoning, the patient should at once be removed from the source of danger, kept lying down covered warmly in a well-ventilated room. Reassure patient and phone the doctor.

Cleaning up domestic air

Domestic air pollution affecting our closest environment cannot fail to harm human beings. Much could be done to prevent or at least reduce it in the name of that blessed word ecology,* recalling that it owes its derivation to the Greek 'oikos', a home. Why should not housewives everywhere as individuals, or in groups, draw up and try to get adopted a Housewives Charter for Clean Domestic Air? Aims and methods might be on the following lines:

Aims

1 To protect the oxygen indoors from robbery and pollution
2 To protect anyone indoors from noxious fumes
3 To improve the outdoor air before it comes indoors

Methods

a No appliance burning gas, solid fuel, coke or paraffin to be used without an adequate vent or chimney
b No smoking indoors, especially in pregnancy, unless in a room set apart for the purpose
c No aerosol pesticides to be used for any purpose indoors
d All do-it-yourself dry cleaning in the home to be done out-of-doors

* Ecology, originally spelt oecology, comes from the Greek 'oikos', a home or dwelling, and 'logos', knowledge. It is defined by the *Shorter Oxford Dictionary* (1950) as 'that branch of biology which deals with the mutual relations between organisms and the environment'.

    e All launderettes offering dry cleaning facilities to their customers to contain well-designed and constructed units providing proper ventilation, as made for dry cleaning establishments

    f To apply pressure to hasten the replacement of internal combustion engines by steam- and electric-powered vehicles for private or public transport

Tailpiece

Canfuls of clean air were made available in Pittsburgh, USA, in January 1970—at a price. A group calling themselves GASP (Group Against Air Pollution) offered tins costing one dollar (about 40p) each and labelled 'Beneficial for all age groups especially children. Do not dilute. Use directly from the can. Open and breathe deeply.' (*Daily Telegraph* 17 January 1970)

REFERENCES

1   SPENCER, T. D. *Ann. Occup. Hyg.*, 5, 251 (1962)
2   CASMEY, W. H. *The Way to the Smokeless City* (C. Griffin, 1926)
3   HILLS, J. B. G., BSC. Personal Communication
4   CARR, DONALD. *The Breath of Life* (Gollancz, 1965)
5   CHANDLER, T. J. *The Air Around Us* (Aldous Books, 1967)
6   MILLS, C. A. *Jour. of Med. Sci.* (March 1960)
7   BRINKMAN, R. *et al. Lancet*, 7325, 133 (1964)
8   STOKINGER, H. E. *et al. Arch. Environ. Health* (10 May 1965)
9   WITHERIDGE, W. N. *et al. Am. Soc. Heat & Vent. Engs.*, 45, 909 (1959)
10   BEDFORD, THOMAS. OBE, DSC., PHD. *Basic Principles of Ventilation and Heating* (Lewis, 1964)
11   GRUEN, L. *Munch. Med. Wocksehr*, 28 (29 March 1962)
12   ROSPA STATISTICS (May 1969)

3

Pollution in the Car

'Transport leaders in Great Britain are sleepwalkers, imitating all the mistakes of the USA.'

LEWIS MUMFORD

The family car, mobile annexe of half the homes in Britain and a higher proportion in some other countries, often goes one better than the family kitchen as a home-made source of CO in a confined space, and has been known to resemble a moving gas chamber for infants and the elderly.

It has been estimated by Professor J. E. Kench that 'an average 1000 cc car puts out about 15 litres per minute of CO and at this rate the air in an ordinary garage could be very dangerous to life in about $2\frac{1}{2}$ minutes'.[1] This underlines the importance of propping open or fastening back the doors before starting up the engine, but, even with this essential precaution, merely taking out and putting away a car may involve inhaling small doses several times daily, and this could reach an unborn child through its expectant mother. From one point of view, it is just as well that so many urban owners leave their cars outside day and night. The siting of garages has an importance too often overlooked. In blocks of flats they should not be incorporated in the basement or ground floor and in most places building regulations require that basement garages must have fire-proof floors which are gas-tight, with independent vents, to prevent the fumes rising and fouling the lower floors, or rising up the lift shafts to foul the upper halls. Converted mews are, perhaps, the worst offenders where whole flats extend over stables turned into garages. Even a direct passageway between a house and its adjacent garage, and certainly a communicating door, have nothing to commend them.

The motoring public seems to be unaware that not only has the MPC of 100 ppm for an eight-hour period been set too high, but is sometimes exceeded in the traffic queues of London and other cities. In Paris, one quarter of the air pollution has been attributed to motor vehicles, and may reach 150 ppm in rush hours. An attempt was made in 1964 to reduce these fumes by fining motorists the equivalent of £4 and up to a week in prison if their vehicles emitted black exhaust fumes. Offenders could also be required to submit their vehicles for inspection to prove that they had been regulated or repaired efficiently. Imagine the outcry if Mrs Barbara Castle had gone as far as this in her efforts to reduce road casualties.

A driver may be so impaired by the inhalation of exhaust fumes, not only from other cars around him but reaching him in a far higher concentration from *his own engine* under conditions which are all too prevalent, that his accident potential may rise to dangerous heights. In the years 1954–6 there were 310 USA Army personnel medically treated in hospital for CO poisoning, and there were ninety-seven deaths due to CO, *not in moving vehicles*. Similarly, in 186 fatal crashes in the USA Air Force, one-third of the victims, in the absence of fire, had blood and tissue levels of carboxyhaemoglobin in excess of 30 per cent at altitudes where they were breathing cabin air in considerable proportion. The comment of the investigators that automobile engines produce CO which accumulates in the absence of adequate ventilation has relevance for every motorist.[2]

How many owner-drivers ever give a thought to the fumes that may seep in to the body of a car from the crank case, the heating system, a leaking gasket or from an exhaust pipe that has rusted into holes from age or corrosion? A well-known motoring correspondent advises that the heater booster should not be used for long periods in city driving, nor the fresh air booster, since they tend to suck in fumes from a vehicle in front or alongside. Furthermore, he considers it is a dangerous mistake to suppose that opening windows while travelling through pure country air can lead to freedom from fumes from one's own leaking exhaust, since an influx of air tends to draw in more fumes.

In 1962, an incident which might have had a fatal outcome was reported in the *Canadian Medical Services Journal*. A Flight Lieutenant of the RCAF Institute of Aviation Medicine, drove a Volkswagen car to work one wintry day with the heater fully on to prevent the windshield from fogging. As a physiologist he was keenly alive to the hazard of CO poisoning, so drove with open windows, but during his forty-five minute drive ten miles through heavy traffic he developed such a severe headache that he suspected CO poisoning. On arrival, laboratory testing of his blood showed a saturation of 22 to 23 per cent and of the heater air, with the engine idling, of 500 ppm. Had the journey lasted thirty-five minutes longer, a rise of blood saturation to 30 per cent could easily have occurred, causing collapse and probably a fatal accident. The futility of trusting to CO indicators under common conditions is stressed by the fact that his indicator (made for use in vehicles and distributed by an automobile club) showed no detectable sign throughout the trip of the colour change which indicates the presence of CO, thus creating a false sense of security.*[3]

Every car owner can take immediate steps to ensure that fumes do not leak into his car from his own faulty exhaust. He can buy one of the long-life replacement silencers that uses special alloy cladding to give full protection against external rusting from road salt, gritty particles, and internal corrosion by exhaust acids and gases. He can fit the special fumes-booster gripping the exhaust pipe now available, and include a regular check for leaking fumes when having his car serviced. Finally, he can follow the example given by Prince Philip when in 1967 he had his Alvis car fitted with a device to cut down noxious emissions on the road.

Compulsory cleaning of internal combustion engines
For many years Los Angeles has headed the list of major cities periodically hit by severe air pollution problems due to temperature inversions† blanketing the area with so-called 'smogs' which, unlike London models, are due to a chemical reaction between ultra-violet radiations from sunlight and noxious fumes from man-made sources. Attempts to identify the culprit became a fiercely contested public issue, and it was not until after the establishment in 1950 of the Los Angeles County Air Pollution Control Laboratory that the chief offender was found to be the internal combustion engine. Since that date, the main objective of State smog authorities has been to clean up the engines, a task considered by some experts about 'a hundred times as difficult as flying a man to the moon'.

Regulations enforcing crankcase vents and specifying permitted amounts of olefin hydrocarbons in motor fuels have been followed

* It has since been found on scientific investigation that such devices fail to function in humidity, or moving vehicles.

† Temperature inversions usually take place at dawn and dusk when rising warm air meets a cold layer above and comes down again. It can often be seen and smelt beside a row of terrace houses whose owners have banked their fires with wrapped sink basket refuse and small coal before retiring.

by others making the use of cleaner devices to reduce the emission of exhaust pollutants compulsory, culminating in July 1969 in the Senate of California sanctioning a bill to ban sales in that State of new vehicles powered by internal combustion engines as from 1 January 1975.

Meanwhile, Federal standards in 1970 in the USA for emission from motor vehicles stood at 180 ppm for hydrocarbons, 100 ppm for CO and 350 ppm for nitrous oxides, with diesel smoke to be reduced to a 'faint plume'. A project known as the Inter-Industry Emission Control Program announced in 1968 that it aimed at reducing emissions of unburned hydrocarbons to 65 ppm of CO to 30 ppm and of nitrogen oxides to 175 ppm. In fact, a spokesman for the American motor industry speaking in 1969 claimed that the main battle had been won, for since 1961 specified emissions had all been reduced and further reductions were planned for later models.

Other authorities seem less well satisfied. According to one chemical expert any emission of nitrous oxide remains largely an unheeded danger, although it should be possible to concentrate on removing the lamentably high concentrations of nitrous oxides produced by the exhaust of diesel engines.[4] The menace of nitrous oxides, over and above their role as potential carcinogens, lies in their habit of combining with ultra-violet rays from sunlight to produce not only nitric oxide but also ozone, now recognized as toxic to plants as well as to man.

Although clear sunlight could hardly have been considered any part of a hazard in the London streets of the past, or in other industrial cities in Britain, it might well become one as the extension of smokeless zones continues to cleanse the air of the smoke that cuts off ultra-violet radiations.

Furthermore, there is mounting evidence of severe environmental damage to soil and vegetation from lead residues derived from the lead alkyls added to petrol to improve the octane rating—the Tiger in the Tank—also contributing to the formation of smogs. Lead tetraethyl (the anti-knock factor in fuel) is very toxic to man. Inhaling the lead from exhaust fumes leads to a far higher concentration in the blood than absorbing it in food.[5] In fact a chemical process company has announced that this could be eliminated at very high cost, and a certain business corporation has claimed that the changes necessary to maintain octane rating without the addition of lead additives would cost the customer as much as a penny a gallon. Presumably they know their public so well that they suppose any customer would rather save a penny a gallon for his pocket than contribute this trifling sum to save himself and his environment from serious harm.

This niggardly approach contrasts strongly with that of seven major American airlines which announced in October 1969 that all their new planes would contain smokeless engines, which would not pollute the air, and cost about £13 million. There were also to be discussions with representatives of the American Air Transport Association on the possibility of all airlines adopting smokeless engines.

Four months later in the House of Commons, Mr Goronwy Roberts, Minister of State at the Board of Trade, stated in a written reply that measurements of smoke pollution caused by aircraft flying into London Airport were to start within six to eight weeks.

Meanwhile, the Swedish Government proposed in 1970 that all cars sold in Sweden from 1971 onwards should be fitted with exhaust cleaners, with compulsory annual inspection of all vehicles to include emissions, and spot checks to be maintained through the year.

Early in 1970 the European Conservation Conference in Strasbourg recommended that all practical means should be used to reduce pollution to a minimum. In particular, the unwanted side effects of the internal combustion engine, jet aircraft and chemicals, should be eliminated as quickly as possible.

A week later Japan announced her intention of placing rigid control on the amounts of CO and other noxious fumes permitted from car exhausts. Sixty-seven inspection stations were being set up to test over sixteen million new and used vehicles. The inspection of the first four million was to start in August.

As even compulsory cleaning up of internal combustion engines resembles mere pecking at a serious problem, what are the alternatives? No less than a wholesale exit of these modern pollution-spitting dragons, and the introduction of less guilty steam cars or, better still, of wholly innocent electric cars. What are the prospects of either? Will steam cars make an entrance as steam trains bow out, will electric buses replace diesel buses, and will electricity finally oust steam, petrol and diesel oil propellants?

The alternatives
An era came to an end on 8 August 1968 when the last steam train on British Railways puffed out of Liverpool with as much sense of an

epic occasion as that of the *Rocket* making its first journey on a mainline passenger service in 1830. It now seems possible that the 1970s may see the beginning of a new era for steam, with the revival of steam cars, which date back to about 1840. These had many early difficulties owing to bulky boilers, the risk of explosions, the consumption of large amounts of water requiring frequent stops to refill, and low volume production. However, by the first decades of the century a car propelled by steam was in production in the USA and had even penetrated Britain. It proved so efficient and likely to become popular, however, that the makers of internal combustion engines stepped in to buy it up, and close down production.

Steam propulsion has not stood still none the less, and there are now modern steam cars with no danger of explosion, as the old boiler has been replaced by a single-tube generator containing only small amounts of water at a time, while it needs only ten gallons of water per 500 miles and burns only one gallon of paraffin oil every twenty-five miles. Committees of the US Senate in 1968 heard a physicist, Dr Robert U. Ayres, outline the present status and advantages of such automobiles, after he had completed an extensive and comprehensive review of present-day steam engines, which had led him to the conclusion that these engines are unquestionably competitive with internal combustion engines.

Britain appears to show only academic interest, but the USA has seen practical attempts to introduce this alternative to petrol and diesel engines, largely as the result of a campaign by William Lear, the millionaire engineer, who believes that all efforts to clean up exhaust gases are doomed to failure. He is working on the production of a steam racing car, as well as offering to supply California at his own expense with a steam bus, and a steam car for the highway patrol.

Although they had previously considered the idea of a steam car impractical, General Motors in 1969 produced two steam-engined cars but found many problems still awaiting solution. Nevertheless whatever the efficiency and cheapness ultimately achieved, steam power could never claim to be entirely pollution or noise free. Yet it has been suggested that the steam car might have a limited innings to fill the estimated thirty-year gap before an acceptable electric car can be in production.

In 1970 Ford and the Thermo Electron Corporation announced in Detroit that they were carrying out a joint five-year programme to develop the commercial applications of a low pollutant steam engine.

Going electric
In 1880 three British professors, having obtained a specimen, wrote a report on 'Mr Edison's new horseshoe lamps'. After a series of careful measurements and determinations of the amount and character of electric current which would be needed to operate it efficiently, they concluded that *'in fact everything is against the electric light* [author's italics] which demands vastly more machinery . . . requires more skilful management, shows more liability to disarrangement and waste, and presents an utter lack of the storage capacity which secures such a vast efficiency, convenience and economy in gas'. Thumbs down for the electric light.

Today, vested interests are equally against the electric car, and in 1969 experts from General Motors and Ford told a Congressional panel that any alternative to the internal combustion engine as a means of propelling cars remained a long way off. However, there seems to be hope that they may be as far off in their calculations as that unbiased seer, H. G. Wells, who foretold in his book *Anticipations*, appearing in 1898, that the first aeroplanes would take the air in the 1950s.

Other eminent authorities in the USA have in fact declared themselves on the side of the anti-polluters. In 1966, Professor Barry Commoner wrote that he considered it 'unlikely that the gasoline driven auto car can long continue to serve as the chief vehicle of urban and suburban transportation, without imposing a health hazard which most of us would be unwilling to accept'. Two years later three professors at Yale University, in medicine and public health, biology, and conservation, respectively, branded the motor car as Public Enemy No. 1 and predicted that 'within 5 to 10 years it would be possible to have an epidemic of lung cancer in a city like Los Angeles'. For many years previously, Lewis Mumford, that enlightened non-Marxist critic of the acquisitive society, had urged the need to replace 'money economy by life economy' without altogether discarding the profit motive, and warned his fellows that they had sacrificed their lives to their cars, forgetting that cities exist for the care and culture of men and not for cars, while stressing the possibility of redesigning these to run electrically.

It is clear then that to save ourselves and our environment, we need not destroy our machines of locomotion but we could do a great deal to prevent them invisibly destroying us by making this radical change in their power supply. In spite of having many powerful enemies and lacking sufficient advocates or funds, electric cars with their small size and ease of parking, no smoke, no smell, lessened fire risk, no imported fuel and most of all *no noxious fumes*, certainly do not lack advantages. It is time all concerned with the ethics and aesthetics, as well as the medical desirability, of removing and not merely reducing the polluting menace of all petrol and oil burning vehicles joined with the National Society for Clean Air in giving un-reserved support to electric traction in all kinds of application and development.

In this connection it is heartening to recall that the Senior Economic Adviser to the Roskill Commission predicted in a paper given at the Third International Road Traffic Conference held in Vienna in 1969 that while it was estimated that by the year AD 2000 eight out of ten British families would be running at least one vehicle, electric cars would be almost universal. How far have they advanced to date?

Progress towards no pollution from cars
There is nothing new in the idea of an electrically powered car. There were electric cabs in London at the start of the century and a few other electric vehicles scattered elsewhere, but development work was hampered by a number of factors, among them the crippling weight of the lead-acid storage battery required to provide adequate power. Another major obstacle was the opposition of American automobile companies, one of which bought the exclusive rights to the patents of a British-designed electric drive motor a few years ago only to consign them to oblivion. Further development therefore ceased, except on delivery vehicles and industrial trucks, where the limita-tions of short range and the length of time required to recharge batteries, were no handicap. By 1966 there were over 40,000 door-to-door electric vans in use in Britain, almost double the number ten years earlier, and far more than in any other country.

By the 1960s the prospects of a market for a second family car restricted to commuting and shopping, combined with the problem of the sale of off-peak electricity, led to a re-investigation by the Electricity Council. Research was sponsored and in 1964 a four-seater electric car powered by a lead-acid battery was displayed at the Electrical Engineers' Exhibition at Earl's Court.

Not to be outdone, Ford had the first electric car to come from a major mass producer on display at the 1967 Motor Show at Earl's Court, insisting that it was a feasible prototype of what could become a practical special-purpose vehicle within ten years, although the chief development engineer for Mercedes Benz passenger cars went on record as saying on the same occasion, '*There is no future whatever* for electric cars at present.' Men heard the same words in 1880, about electric light.

Delegates at the 1968 annual meeting of the Swedish local traffic agencies expressed the hope that buses operated by fuel cells of the type used in American space-ships (perhaps the most immediately useful item to emerge from the whole venture) would become practicable in a few years.

At the Sixth International Power Sources Symposium held in Brighton in September 1968, engineers discussed how fuel cell/ secondary battery, and diesel engine/secondary hybrids might eventually displace the conventional diesel engines at present in use all over the world. In November 1969 the Chairman of the Metropolitan Transportation Authority announced at a Symposium on Air Pollution and Respiratory Diseases held in New York that two electrically operated buses were to go into use in Manhattan on an experimental basis, working on short cross-town services and recharging batteries at stations maintained at each end.

Development work continues to concentrate on trying to raise the power-to-weight ratio by the use of different metals in storage batteries, by battery fuel cell hybrids, and by various types of fuel cells converting electro-chemical reactions directly into electricity. Increased efforts in this field were forecast by Professor J. Kolbus-zewski at the annual meeting of the Public Transport Association in Brighton in 1969.

Suggesting that the ultimate goal of fuel cell application may be in the electric vehicle, experts summarized the situation at the end of 1969 as follows:

'Fuel cell technology has progressed to the stage where electro-chemistry can reach applications which exploit one or more of the virtues of the fuel cell. Several companies have specific programmes aimed at developing and overcoming the engineering problems of producing integrated power-plants. The fuel cell, judged by its past and present progress, will achieve a wider range of markets than at present and *in the ultimate it will compete with mains electrical supplies and internal combustion engine generators.*'[6] (Author's italics.)

It begins to look as if the 'mess of wattage', to misquote one of its

engineers, might in the end mean the loss of heritage by the automobile industry. The electric car is now a feasible proposition. The
future holds fresh encouragement for all who are passionately
involved in diminishing air pollution because they are involved in
mankind.

Perils of a passenger
Since there is a tendency in a moving vehicle for its own fumes to
be sucked in through open windows or any other aperture, it is best
to sit in the front seats of diesel buses with rear engines. In station
wagons, where the eddy currents set up by the vacuum in the rear of a
fast moving vehicle are particularly apt to suck in the engine's own
exhaust fumes, rear seats are best avoided. In the opinion of a medical
expert most car sickness is attributable to fumes, not motion.[7] In
fact, it seems best to avoid being a passenger at all! Too few owners
take the trouble to check the integrity of exhaust pipes, although these
are usually made of such perishable material that they are not likely
to outlast a year's use, especially after exposure to the corroding
effects of salt and grit.

Anyone dismissing these inhalations lightly is invited to consider
the conclusions reached in a paper published in the Archives of
Environmental Health in May 1966. Chronic exposure of experimental animals to various concentrations (no higher than those to
which many motorists unwittingly expose their children) of exhaust-
air mixtures resulted in significant biological effects indicating increased susceptibility to pulmonary infection and chronic disease
during the later half of life, and decreased fertility and survival rate
of infant mice. This exposure caused a stress response, increased lead
concentrations in bone and an increase in the amount of non-
functional and abnormal lung tissue. The investigators considered
that further studies were indicated.[8] These findings imply that
taking time and thought to prevent exhaust fumes being disseminated
inside a car would be worthwhile for everyone.

Combining CO with alcohol or cigarettes
Some six years before Mrs Barbara Castle succeeded in reducing
road casualties by bringing in breathalyser tests, investigators of the
alcohol problem in Germany had found, during work on fatalities
following the continuous action of CO on humans (and mice) under
the influence of alcohol, that the lethal cases showed considerably

lower levels of carboxyhaemoglobin than those without alcohol. The investigators summed up their conclusions in the presumption that the booster (synergistic) effect also plays a part in small doses of CO and alcohol and may even be the cause of impaired efficiency in traffic, while admitting that they have no exact evidence on this point.[9] But the idea is beginning to spread that a number of traffic accidents may be as directly or indirectly attributable to errors of judgement in drivers affected by CO from whatever source, as in those affected by alcohol.

Heavy cigarette smokers have been found to carry from 4 to 8 per cent of carboxyhaemoglobin, reducing the oxygen content of their blood to the equivalent of that on first reaching an altitude of 7000 feet. In commenting on this finding, in 1966, Mr Ross A. Macfarland of Harvard University stressed that as the initial reaction of CO consists of lowered attention, difficulty in concentrating and lethargy, additional CO entering the body of the car from *its own* exhaust fumes, when the driver is already deficient in oxygen due to smoking, might have very serious implications for road safety.

REFERENCES

1   KENCH, J. E. *Manchester Univ. Med. School Gazette*, Vol. 37, No. 1 (January 1958)
2   *Army Medical Research & Nut. Lab. Report*, 261 (1 September 1961)
3   MACNAMARA, W. D. *Med. Serv. Jour.* (Canada, June 1962)
4   CARR, DONALD. *The Breath of Life* (Gollancz, 1965)
5   KENCH, J. E. *Manchester Univ. Med. School Gazette*, Vol. 37, No. 1. (January 1958)
6   *New Scientist* (13 November 1969)
7   RANDOLPH, THERON. *Anns. of Allergy*, 19 (June 1961)
8   HUETER, F. G. *et al. Arch. Environ. Health*, 12, No. 5 (May 1966)
9   MALLACH, H. J. *et al. Arzneimittelforsch.* (11 November 1961)

4

Tobacco—The Personal Pollution

'Smoking is the most intensive form of air pollution
anyone can submit themselves to.'
                    PROFESSOR PATRICK LAWTHER

Oxygen deficiency is not the only disability suffered by
smokers. Far from it. Warning posters and school lectures are designed to make young flesh creep, and journalists repeatedly publicize
the wider hazards. But there is little decrease in the sale of tobacco.
Why is this?

According to a report of 1968 the Government collected in duty
about £1000 million from taxes on tobacco of the £1500 million odd
spent annually by the British public on tobacco products. Might not
this be the basic reason? A former Chancellor of the Exchequer said
in Parliament in 1957, 'We at the Treasury do not want too many
people to stop smoking.' Yet the experts consider that the alarming
figures for lung cancer and coronary deaths will continue to rise
unless a great many people give up smoking, and also that one of the
reasons for the post-war pressures for higher pay has been the
increased price of tobacco, since tobacco is a must for some twenty
million of us.

So the Treasury continues to clutch its money bags stuffed with
tobacco duty to the figure of some £1000 million annually, while
handing out a paltry £100,000 to the Ministry of Health to pay
for a token attempt to discourage people from buying tobacco. This
looks like a highly profitable transaction. When one adds to the debit
account the statement by Lord Cohen of Birkenhead, President of
the General Medical Council, that 'cigarette smoking is now a major
cause of both illness and death in Britain, causing an estimated ten
per cent of the yearly deaths' with all that this entails in suffering
and loss of life and livelihood to family and country, it begins to look
more like blood money than legitimate excise.

As the Chief Medical Officer at the Ministry of Health, Sir George

Godber courageously announced in his Annual Report in 1968, 'These are the sacrifices made to a lethal folly.'[1] How much longer is our tragic inability to look unpleasant facts in the face to continue? How much longer must our hospitals and nursing homes be filled with patients dying from preventable diseases? Preventable, that is, only if they could be persuaded to give up their 'lethal folly'.

Why not spend some of the millions devoted to research into the present unknown fundamental nature of cancer on combating at least this one well-established correlate of lung cancer and bronchitis, simply by guiding smokers into less suicidal and inhumane habits? Yes, inhumane. What other habit among civilized people is not only offensive but definitely harmful to others around the habituated person, and even to his or her unborn child?

The writer of an introduction to a book by a fellow physician on smoking, published in 1958, could state that 'smoking by one individual, though often disagreeable to others, *has not been shown to carry any risk for others who are non-smokers*'.[2] (Author's italics.) This comforting assumption is no longer valid; indeed it never was, for in 1944 Dr F. L. Wood pointed out that a non-smoker absorbs enough of the nicotine freed in the air of any smoky ill-ventilated room to develop coronary disease,[3] and in 1967 Dr J. C. Harris, of the Imperial Cancer Research Institute, in a summary of his work, stated that he had induced lung cancer in mice by making them breathe cigarette smoke.[4] They were smoked at, as non-smokers are. *They did not smoke cigarettes themselves.*

Two years later Professor Lynne Reid and a colleague at the Institute of Diseases of the Chest in London showed that rats exposed to the smoke from five, ten or twenty cigarettes or the equivalent in cigar smoke, developed in a mere six weeks changes in the goblet (mucus-producing) cells of their lung passages resembling those in human sufferers of chronic bronchitis.[5]

These findings clearly endorse the strong suspicion that having to spend evening after evening in the smoky atmosphere of a public house pushes the publican to the bottom of the life expectancy ladder. We may bite our nails with no harm to any but ourselves, but only a hermit in a desert can smoke without detriment to others, and any unprejudiced observer must agree with the medical officer of health who asserted that 'No one has the right to poison the air that someone else breathes.'

Respiratory and cardiac cases undergoing treatment in hospital may be subjected to unremitting tobacco smoke from fellow patients, and frequently smoke themselves, since this is permitted even in the medical wards of renowned teaching hospitals. Such disregard of the unqualified opinion of the experts can do little to teach, much less impress on doctors and nurses in training the general hazards to health involved, quite apart from the damaging effect on the sick in their care.

There are, however, slight signs of a stirring of official consciences in this field. In 1967 an Australian hospital reported that the results of admitting patients to a non-smoking ward had clearly demonstrated the benefits. Patients with respiratory conditions had previously been allowed to smoke while receiving advanced treatment. Staff from other wards commented on the clean air and the relative absence of night coughing, and all the thirty-six male patients involved were in favour of the non-smoking regulations, which were strictly enforced and extended for these patients to everywhere in the hospital. This was especially the case with the heavy smokers, who found shared abstinence easier to bear, and all felt better for the deprivation by the date of discharge.

The fact that the innovation was so readily accepted surely has wider implications. In the words of the medical officer publishing the report: 'Is it unreasonable to suppose that the notion of this kind of ward should spread throughout hospitals in general?'[6]

The Methodist Hospital of Indiana had already made a unique three-year study of an in-patient smoking control among its patients and reached the conclusion that patients had been helped 'to sustain control of their smoking habits after discharge at a reduced or zero level'.[7]

Perhaps the invidious situation is best summed up in the words of the executive board of the United Nations World Health Organization in Geneva in its request issued in 1970 that members attending meetings should refrain from smoking—'No organization devoted to the promotion of health can be neutral in this matter.'[8]

Many would wish to add 'nor any organization devoted to the promotion of anti-pollution'.

At least six places are now recognized where non-smokers are at risk from smokers. These are on the road; in the womb; in the forest; in any aircraft; in ships at sea; in any smoke-laden room.

1 Smoking heavily raises the level of CO in the blood. This, added to the level of CO due to breathing in fumes from traffic or even his

own exhaust, may cause symptoms in a driver leading to a fatal accident involving the lives of others.

2 Smoking during pregnancy can so affect the unborn child that for its further life it may be disabled in lesser or greater degree as a consequence.[10] Indeed, this could also be true of 'passive smoking' through a husband who smokes heavily.

3 Forest fires started by cigarette ends have caused many deaths as well as great economic loss. In British Columbia the Government took this so seriously that in 1967 a Non-Smoking Day was proclaimed for 31 May by Order in Council.[11] This was aimed at encouraging people not to smoke, not only on that day but thereafter, in the interest of health as well as for the protection of their valuable forests.

4 In aeroplanes, pressurized today to roughly the atmospheric pressure at 5000 feet, passengers already suffer a slight deprivation of oxygen. To have smokers pollute their available air with tobacco fumes is to pile Ossa on Pelion, to say nothing of the distress it causes to most of the non-smokers shut up with them in this very restricted space. Moreover, fires are an ever present hazard from careless smokers, and it is significant that smoking is not permitted at the moments of greatest danger, i.e. at take-off and landing. Why not all the time passengers are air-borne? There are always stops where smokers could light up on land, in the open.

5 The chief cause of fires at sea, according to a director of Cunard, is cigarette ends. Incidentally, the lack of any indoor accommodation free from ash-trays and the spiralling smoke from the smouldering duty-free cigarettes can do a great deal to spoil the pleasantest voyage for a non-smoker.

6 There is a great difference among non-smokers in their susceptibility to nausea in smoke-filled rooms. A well-known non-smoking physician always complained of palpitation, headache and insomnia after attending medical meetings in Munich, for doctors are often heavy smokers off duty. The National Society of Non-Smokers has evidence that its members and probably many thousands of others suffer in this or in an even more unpleasant way.

Why tobacco is dangerous
The smoke of burning tobacco is an obvious nuisance, in that it stains and fouls paint, furnishings and clothing, to say nothing of the damage and risk due to smouldering dog-ends. Its real menace for

man, however, lies in factors only revealed on scientific analysis. These include gases and volatile tars, methyl (or wood) alcohol, benzopyrenes, pyridine, selenium, arsenic and nicotine.[12] The amount of carbon monoxide produced in smoking one cigarette is alone enough to cause symptoms. It is believed that the methyl alcohol may lead to amblyopia causing temporary blindness in some people and to total blindness in diabetics who smoke, because it is cumulative in action. Pyridine, a coal tar derivative, selenium derived from the combination of the cigarette paper with the benzopyrenes, also arsenic, are all under suspicion as carcinogens, responsible especially for cancer of the lungs, mouth and oesophagus. Arsenic is also considered responsible for the skin poisoning of chronic smokers, and may be a factor of some importance in eczema. Smokers frequently present a discoloured and wrinkled skin, to the profit of those concerned to keep these drawbacks at bay by cosmetics. In food the legally permitted limit in the USA for arsenic is 1·43 ppm, but investigators in 1937 found levels in tobacco fifty times as high from sprays used on the crop.

As for nicotine, this poison is present in such quantity and is so powerful that just one cigarette lowers the temperature of the fingers and toes by over five degrees through constriction of the arteries, which also occurs in the retina of the eye and persists after the cigarette is finished.[13] For the same reason less oxygen gets through to the cortex of the brain, which may cause mental distress, and there may be clotting of the narrow passages of the terminal arteries of the legs leading to an agonizingly painful condition known as Buerger's disease, which can result in gangrene if not treated and smoking abandoned. In disease of the coronary arteries, when this has reached the stage of causing the acute pain in heart or stomach, characteristic of this trouble, it is often too late to be reversed.

Nicotine also paralyses the tiny waving hairlike masses of cilia which work to scoop up any foreign particles breathed in so they can be coughed up and ejected, or be swallowed. This may mean an inability to reject TB or other microbes, impurities and carcinogens in polluted air. Furthermore, the nicotine content of nine cigarettes a day is enough to interfere with the blood supply to the reproductive system, especially in women.[14] In addition, the normal resting pulse rate of around seventy-two may be raised by as much as twenty-eight beats, or on an average by ten beats per minute, thus upsetting its steady rhythm and introducing a stop-and-go-beat. The faster a cigarette is smoked, the more nicotine is produced, although only one-third of this goes into the mouth to be absorbed by the smoker; the other two-thirds goes into the air to be 'passively smoked' by anyone else present.*[15]

Other ill effects of nicotine result from its indirect action on the adrenal glands. Their output of hormones is boosted up to fifty per cent by heavy smoking which releases sugar into the circulation, giving the 'lift' of the first few puffs. But the excess of adrenalin in the blood raises the pressure and lowers the blood sugar. This may lead to just another cigarette for the sake of the short preliminary 'lift', and so *ad infinitum*, or to a craving for sugar which has its own ill effects. This is likely to cause a diabetes-like condition and/or a rise in the businessman's nightmare, cholesterol, the most commonly suggested causal agent of arteriosclerosis.[16]

Those who prefer to believe that these are disabilities suffered in the main only by the humbler hospital patient, would do well to consider the case of the late King George VI, who was a heavy cigarette smoker. He ran the gamut of constrictions of the arteries of his legs, corrected by operation; cancer of the lung, partly removed by surgeons; then, mercifully, death in his sleep from a coronary. Though he escaped the terminal sufferings of lung cancer, he paid the price as fully as the poorest of his people. They may all have been smokers themselves, but one cannot help wondering if any of the eminent doctors who attended the Royal person ever tried by example or persuasion to wean him from his dangerous habit before it wrecked his health and claimed his life at fifty-six.

It is cheering to recall that there have been men at the top who have listened to and acted on such advice, to their own great benefit. 'That will be your last cigarette,' a doctor is reported to have said to President Johnson as he lit up in the ambulance taking him to hospital after a heart attack in 1955. It was. Like his predecessor President Eisenhower, he stopped smoking on his physician's advice.

Fifty years ago a colonel in the RAMC asserted that: 'In heart and nervous disorders nicotine is poison, and medical men are well aware of this, but do not take a firm stand as it would make them un-

---

* These facts were published over twenty-five years ago but have been largely disregarded. By contrast, as soon as it was discovered that computers may be damaged by smoke and ash, these *valuable machines* were protected by 'No Smoking' notices.

popular.'[17] Fortunately, this attitude has been overcome and investigations into the dangers in connection with lung cancer were reviewed very authoritatively by the Royal College of Physicians in 1962. Their report was coupled with an appeal for decisive Government action to curb the rising consumption of tobacco.[18] Owing to its ambivalent attitude referred to in an earlier paragraph, the Government has done little to implement this appeal. It is noteworthy that Lord (then Sir Robert) Platt, President of the Royal College of Physicians, and Chairman of the Committee responsible for the report, had himself been a heavy smoker until 1954. Persuaded by the evidence presented of the dangers of the habit, he gave it up from that date.

It remains for other and lesser medical men to set the same example. Accustomed to exact attention to their advice in other health matters, they could, if they would, use their authority to advantage and speak out. No one with the good fortune to be present will forget the involuntary outburst of applause for the Professor of Medicine at Cape Town University, Dr J. F. Brock, when in the course of a lecture on 'Nature, nurture and stress' at the Summer School of 1963 he told a packed audience that 'Smoker's bravado' (the you-can't-frighten-me-syndrome) was the intellectual refuge of stupid men.

The fallacies of filters, herbal or therapeutic cigarettes and snuff-taking

Naturally the big tobacco companies have been exploring every possibility of producing a 'safe' cigarette. Taking their cue from the well-publicized immunity to lung cancer of Yemeni Jews living in Israel, who always smoke through a filter, they have suggested that filter tips to cigarettes remove the danger. There are two fallacies here. The Yemenis do not smoke cigarettes but narghile pipes, and the smoke is drawn through water which acts successfully as a filter.[19] Any other type merely takes out the coarser particles leaving the finer ones of smoke and the aerosols. This may actually lead to a larger number of smaller particles managing to reach the lungs simply because they are not blocked in their passage by the larger ones. As Dr Donald Frederickson, who conducts New York's Smoking Control Programme, has put it, 'There is no evidence that filter cigarettes significantly reduce the health risks of smoking.' In any case, a filter capable of removing all the harmful elements would reduce the pleasure to the level of sucking a dummy, and the fact that the narghile pipe gives satisfaction may be due to the effort that is required to draw smoke through it which ensures inhalation and consequently a more effective absorption of the remaining narcotic content.

In an attempt to promote lettuce smoking, the outer leaves of lettuce, which contain no nicotine, have been rolled so as to resemble tobacco after drying, shredding and curing chemically. But in the USA this venture was a failure after one year of promising sales in 1966-7. The brand name Bravo and the rights to the process were sold in 1968 to new owners who are reported to have experimented with different flavours, calling their product Triumph. It is to be hoped that this will not lead to a triumph in sales, since lighting and burning the paper or any vegetable material must, like a small-scale bonfire, produce the benzopyrenes which are carcinogens. As Professor Alexander Haddow, the cancer expert, has emphasized, 'The "safe" cigarette is wishful thinking.' The same stricture must apply to those labelled therapeutic.

As for those refugees from cigarettes who turn to pipes and cigars, they will draw little comfort from the recent revelation that these forms of smoking increase the chance of developing cancer of the kidney by up to twelve times.[20]

There are signs of a move, especially among the young and trendy to replace smoking by taking snuff. Raleigh and his followers smoked pipes, but in Britain by the eighteenth century smoking was mostly confined to male company, and only snuff was used by the fashionable and when ladies were present. Even Dr Johnson—no purist in personal habits—followed suit, avowing that 'to be sure it is a shocking thing blowing smoke out of our mouths into other people's mouths, eyes, and noses'. Later the Crimean heroes came back with Turkish cheroots and popularized the cigarette in England, though it was common in America and Southern Europe before their day.

In 1967 there were said to be about 500,000 snuff-takers in Britain and the President of the Society of Snuff Grinders, Blenders, Purveyors and Connoisseurs has stated that more young people are buying snuff, perhaps because of the cancer warnings and in the belief that the *British Medical Journal* had indicated that it is harmless. This seems to be based on a report in that journal in 1951 that the easiest way to stop smoking is to substitute snuff-taking. This may be, but the belief that it is harmless must be qualified. Snuff, being a form of ground tobacco, contains from 1 to 3 per cent nicotine which is readily absorbed by the mucous membranes of the nose and nasal passages. If taken to excess it could reach the level of that absorbed by smoking. On the other hand consuming 1 oz monthly would only equal from 3 to 19 mg, about as much as if one cigarette were inhaled.[21]

The only way to deal with any habit, much less with an addiction, is by persuasion and example. Clearly this must begin among school children who are at the critical age for the formation of habits, good or bad.

A survey carried out in this country in the 1950s among 3479 young people (1797 boys, 1682 girls) aged from ten to eighteen years from six schools near London revealed that most early smokers were found among the least intelligent. Probably cultural patterns have an important bearing on the results, since it was found that those in public and grammar schools start later and smoke less than those in secondary modern schools. However that may be, it was noted that 80 per cent of the boys had become regular smokers within two years of their first cigarette.[22] For young smokers or prospective smokers, too prone to smoker's bravado, a more off-putting prospect than lung cancer at fifty may be that of no teeth at thirty. In a bio-statistical analysis of patients over an eight-year span, investigators reporting in the *Journal of the American Dental Association* found that there was heightened degeneration and destruction of gums, bone and connective tissue among cigarette smokers, often leading to loss of teeth fifteen years younger than among non-smokers.

Cigarette smoking offers at best a fleeting and ever diminishing satisfaction, and it can be a heart-warming consolation for parents-to-be who give it up to know that, by the self-denial and discipline undoubtedly required, they have avoided exposing their child during its pre-natal life to the harmful influence of their self-destructive habit.

Although the physiological aspect has received the fuller attention of researcher, the psychological has not been neglected. A report from Harvard University to the New York Academy of Sciences[23] in 1966 gave an analysis of personality traits characteristic of smokers and non-smokers in nursing, high schools and colleges which is likely to make many blush to admit that they are smokers. It was found that smokers tend to be more extroverted, gregarious, outgoing and sociable. All pleasing attributes, it may be agreed. But what of the following additional traits? Smokers are more disagreeable and less good-natured, less trusting, less self-reliant, less dependable, less persevering as well as less orderly, mannerly and refined in their person and habits. It begins to look as if the image so studiously built up by the advertisers may be entirely misleading. The Chief Medical Officer at the Ministry of Health, Sir George Godber, seems to have been fully justified when he wrote: 'For commercial purposes and advantage, cigarette smoking is constantly presented to the young as a glamorous and rewarding activity rather than the costly, dirty and damaging habit it is.' How is this false image best countered?

The rewards of giving up smoking
The classic studies of Bradford Hill and R. Doll (who in 1950 first demonstrated the association of smoking with lung cancer) on the smoking habits of 40,000 doctors revealed that among those who had given up smoking for ten years or more the incidence of lung cancer fell to about its level among those who had never smoked.[23] So for heavy smokers who give up this poison, the reward may be very great. Not only has it been established that 'the chain can be broken at the smoking stage, and lung cancer prevented', according to Dr Peter Alexander of the Chester Beatty Research Institute, but a minor benefit also follows. In the experience of a fishing expert he will get better luck when angling, at least for mullet, who are fastidiously put off by any bait with the faintest smell of nicotine from the stained fingers of a smoker. On the other hand, bringing up phlegm daily and persistently is a warning that you are particularly likely to get lung cancer. If you heed this warning you will give up smoking immediately.[24]

According to a statement by Surgeon General William Steward, some nineteen million Americans have given up cigarettes since a government report, which gave scientific evidence showing cigarette smoking to be a 'serious health hazard' linked with cancer and bronchitis was published.

A few months later this was followed by the offer of some companies in the USA of cheaper life insurance policies to non-smokers, amounting in some cases to a reduction of up to 6 per cent of the premium, the qualifying proviso being that no cigarettes had been smoked for a year. One of the companies made a further distinction in raising the premium of smoking policy holders with lung or heart disease above that of similarly affected non-smokers. This seems a highly practical way of encouraging adults to give up smoking and should give other countries a lead.

A study of some 3500 students at the University of Illinois published in 1967 showed that over 59 per cent of those with low marks and who did not join in college activities were smokers, while those with high marks included only 16·7 per cent of smokers. This supports Dr E. J. Grace in his view that smoking is a habit that will persist until men and women are 'more adequately prepared mentally to cope with our complex civilization' and reminds us that the example of parent, doctor or educator can wield a great influence over those who do not resent being educated. Indeed, the value of non-smoking by way of example was stressed by the World Conference on Smoking and Health held in New York in September 1967, when at the first meeting of its kind—organized by the American Cancer Society—487 scientists, educators, physicians and government officials from thirty-eight countries met to discuss the problem.

Prevention had also been the object behind the government anti-smoking campaign in Holland which sent letters to the parents of 300,000 children in elementary schools, urging them to stop smoking in the interest of their children. This brings us back to the findings of the World Congress on Smoking, namely that non-smoking by example carries the greater prospect of success. So, in this matter of immeasurable importance, it is up to parents at home, teachers in schools and colleges, and leaders of fashion in the field of cultural habits to set a new standard of socially acceptable behaviour and to strike out into the exciting world of non-conformity.

Every cigarette smoked is a concession to a conformity which kills. Make no mistake about that. Our tobacco-tyrannized society demands rebels and revolution. No need for barricades or stoning police. What is needed is the courage to abstain. Who better than the protesting young to lead the way in fighting this personal tyranny? This calls for far more valour and originality than any long-haired conformity in dress and behaviour. The one-upmanship of 'Look, no hands' on the bicycle could grow up into 'Look, no fag in the mouth' and this could in turn develop into a social pressure to give up tobacco altogether—as spitting has been given up in living memory.

This could be achieved if the stars of stage, TV and film were to make a public stand against a futile fashion. It would do much to justify the fantastic money and adulation they now enjoy, and could but brighten their image. Who ever saw a Romeo with a gasper on his lip? One hears the plea that there is some social value implying the existence of some esoteric cult of grace and graciousness to guest and colleague connected with cigarette smoking. How is it that Arabs earned their traditionally high reputation for impeccable hospitality and generosity as hosts without them? Can it be that we in the West are so little trained in self-discipline that we cannot feel at ease unless our hand and lip are occupied? Why not offer raisins and peanuts or even celery sticks instead of what Dr Donald Gould has christened 'cancer sticks'? Why do we remain chained to this convention for breaking the ice? How did people in the pre-Raleigh centuries manage without our sop to sociability?

Meanwhile, as we wait for these new Dantons to arise, we must surely give our support to all who point the way to ridding ourselves of this cruel tyranny. From his unique experience of its effects, Mr Ronald Raven, senior surgeon at the Royal Cancer Hospital, has stated categorically, 'Tobacco must go.' This ultimate aim can only be made to succeed by concerted action in a number of directions, such as the following:

1 a. Government restriction on sales and advertising in any medium—the Irish Government has already torpedoed an incentive scheme in the Republic.

b. Restrictions on smoking in all public transport, including aircraft and ships at sea, to limited and isolated accommodation, and also in all public buildings such as hospitals, cinemas, restaurants and shops. It has been suggested that audiences would not accept 'No Smoking' notices in cinemas. This is nonsense. They do, because there is no alternative, in Spain, Sweden, Finland, France, the USSR and some places in the USA, while in parts of New York it is also prohibited in the Subway. Even in Britain this ban is accepted in most London theatres and concert halls, but we still lag far behind other countries in this respect. The booby prize must be awarded, however, to the Cape Town suburban trains, where in long Pullman carriages each carefully labelled 'Whites' or 'Non-Whites', a few seats in each are marked 'Do not smoke'. Souls must be segregated—smoke need not.

2 Setting up many more Non-Smoking Clinics, and starting a

group on the lines of Alcoholics Anonymous, to be called perhaps Tobacco Taboo, for smokers ready to help each other to reach the status of non-smokers.

That public restrictions on harmful habits can be effective is shown by the decrease and eventual disappearance of spitting. In 1915 when spitting, general and unrestricted, spread broadcast active cultures of tubercle bacilli to float in the air as the sputum dried, the annual death rate in Britain from TB was 1100 per million. In 1955 when spitting in public places had been banned for years, and social custom frowned on the habit in private, the figure had dropped to 672. Obviously it is easier to control and eventually eradicate a habit which is merely anti-social than one which also gives pleasure to the habituated. A non-smoker who lives minus morning cough, spoilt palate, stained fingers, bad breath and the rest, feels no deprivation. He may even smugly congratulate himself on money saved by his ability to say 'No' to a senseless convention. For a smoker, to give up the illusory well-being which cloaks the danger is a very different thing. It means a struggle to free himself from a habit to which he is devoted if not already addicted, and in the technical sense he needs all the help he can be given.

The clear duty of any Government with a sufficient majority to defy temporary unpopularity is to take the following steps:

1 a. Forbid by law any advertising in any medium which suggests by no matter what psychologically subtle means that a person may gain anything in pleasure or prestige by putting into his or her mouth a proved habit-forming poison which will in fact do nothing but steal away health and shorten life.

b. Remove from unsupervised public access the vending machines which, in blatant defiance of a Government Order of 1933, make the open direct sale of cigarettes easy to those under sixteen.

c. Extend no-smoking regulations to all public transport and other confined places of public assembly, except in separate accommodation provided for smokers.

Any Government putting these reforms into effect would perform a unique public service ensuring for it a lasting place in history.

2 The first clinic for the treatment of smokers trying to turn into non-smokers was opened in 1957 by Dr Lennox Johnston, but there are still only about one hundred now open in Great Britain. At Harwell Atomic Station hypnosis is being tested out to help scientists there to give up smoking, and the medical officer carrying out the

treatment has estimated that 60 per cent will overcome their habit.

In spite of the suicidal bent of the nicotine addict, clinics could usefully be opened at key points over the country to try out different treatments. The proposal to spend valuable resources of skilled staff and buildings in this way might not be readily accepted in face of the competing demands from other early diagnostic procedures such as cervical smears. It might, however, be pointed out that this was also said of now well-established preventive resources such as VD clinics, and it could hardly be disputed that success would pay off heavily in terms of useful lives saved and disability prevented.

Another and harrowing aspect of the matter is the terminal suffering of the victim of lung cancer which few smokers are aware of and none foresee until too late. Anyone who knows the cruelty of these sufferings must resolve to rescue the potential victims in spite of themselves. This can only be successfully attempted on a national scale.

3 The National Society of Non-Smokers* formed in 1920 counts many eminent people among its members but it needs more supporters and funds to extend its campaign 'to uphold the rights of non-smokers, to curb smoking in public places, to liberate slaves of smoking, and to save youth from being enslaved.'

Reckoning the cost and the obligation
We shall expect howls of rage at the cost of implementing some or all of these proposals. Objections may be expected from those who see such problems only in terms of finance rather than in terms of health and lives saved, but, even to them, it can be shown that the profit and loss would probably balance, because money expended by one government department would be saved by another. The huge sums needed would be recouped from the equally huge sums saved by the government departments and public transport in the form of lowered expenditure on repairs and refurbishing necessitated by the use of tobacco.

There would also follow a large reduction in the number of fires with a corresponding reduction in losses to insurance companies and calls upon fire brigades. The initial and running cost of clinics to help smokers to become non-smokers, would be balanced by a

* Address: 125, West Dumpton, Ramsgate.

generous recompense from the reduction of disabilities giving rise to claims for sick benefit. These disabilities cause the loss of about a hundred million working days in a year, fill hospital beds and outpatient departments and require the provision of pensions for the widows and orphans of men lost to family and employer in their prime. In addition, since tobacco is imported, there would be a favourable adjustment to our balance of payments.

Millions of pounds have been contributed by a compassionate public for research into the causes and cure of cancer. Now this same public has been told in no uncertain words what is causing some frequently occurring forms of cancer and how this can be prevented. 'Tobacco is the cause, and must go completely,' say the most eminent researchers. How can anyone continue to ignore the undeniable evidence and the authoritative advice without making a mockery not only of the devoted researchers but of himself? Giving up smoking and helping others to give up or never to begin are definite contributions that we can all make towards lessening our personal pollution of the air, so lessening the vaster problem of man's pollution of his planet.

There will be many battles before we can hope to triumph, but overcome we must, if only for the sake of the unborn to whom we owe a happier and healthier legacy than the tyranny of tobacco.

REFERENCES

1 'On the State of the Public Health', HMSO Annual Report of the C.M.O. of Ministry of Health (1968)
2 McCURDY, ROBERT, H. B., CHB., DPH. *Smoking, Lung Cancer And You* (Linden Press, London, 1958)
3 WOOD, F. L., MD. *What You Should Know About Tobacco* (Zondervan, 1944)
4 HARRIS, R. J. C. *et al. BMJ*, 4, 637–41 (16 December 1967)
5 REID, LYNNE *et al. BMJ* (2 January 1969)
6 LLOYD, F. T. *et al. Hosp. Management*, 193, 6 (June 1967)
7 SANGSTER, J. F. *Medical Officer* (1967)
8 VALIC, F. *et al. Arch. Za Hig. RADA*, Vol. 5. (1954)
9 WOOD, F. L., MD. *What You Should Know About Tobacco* (Zondervan, 1944)
10 MONTAGU, PROFESSOR ASHLEY. *Life Before Birth* (Longmans, 1964)
11 JOULES, H. *The Health Education Journal*, 1572 (September 1956)
12 WOOD, F. L., MD. *Tobacco* (Zondervan, 1944)
13 *Ibid.*
14 *Ibid.*

15   *Ibid.*
16   KERSHBAUM, DR A. *Jour. Am. Med. Assoc.*, Vol. 203, 275 (1968)
17   WOOD, F. L., MD. *Tobacco* (Zondervan, 1944)
18   *Smoking and Health, Report by Royal College of Physicians* (Pitman Medical Publishing, 1962)
19   MANN, H. K. *Lancet*, 1, 392 (1955)
20   BENNINGTON, J. *et al. Cancer*, Vol. 21, 1069 (1968)
21   *British Medical Journal*, 1, 1155, (1951)
22   *British J. Prev. Soc. Med.*, 13, 1–4 (London School H. and T. D., 1959)
23   HILL, BRADFORD A. and DOLL, R. *BMJ*, 1, 399 (1964)
24   RIMINGTON, J., MD. *BMJ*, Vol. 1, 732 (1968)

5

The Importance of Being Parents

'In the dark womb where I began
My mother's life made me a man.'

JOHN MASEFIELD

Balzac once remarked that the goddess presiding over maternity was chance. This presiding goddess can, in fact, be the expectant mother herself, although to reach this high rank she needs much more than the natural desire to do the best she can for her future offspring. She needs clear ideals and some acquired knowledge on how to choose habits of outlook and living that will achieve this desire. These are necessarily formed before conception takes place and are best begun long before.

At a Symposium on Biology and Ethics held in 1968, Sir Alan Parkes drew up one article of a Declaration of Human Obligations, presenting a code of ethics any parent-to-be should be proud to follow. This stated:

'It is an obligation of men and women . . .

1 Not to produce unwanted children.

2 Not to take a substantial risk of begetting a mentally or physically defective child.

3 Not to produce children, because of irresponsibility or religious observance, merely as a by-product of sexual intercourse.

4 To plan the number and spacing of births in the best interest of mother, child and the rest of the family.

5 To give the best possible mental and physical environment to the child during its formative years, and to produce children, therefore, only in the course of an affectionate and stable relationship between man and woman.

6 However convinced the individual may be of his or her superior qualities, not for this reason to produce children in numbers which, if equalled by everyone, would be demographically catastrophic.'

With these aims accepted and on their way to becoming established, we might indeed be on the road to the new world visualized by Middleton Murry when he referred to 'the tenderly begotten, tenderly nurtured child [who] is the substance of which a new world can be produced'. How can parents-to-be best live up to this code, which is not only ethical, but practicable?

All these clauses presuppose contraception. To take or not to take The Pill—that is the question. Today, the immediacy of the answer hovers over everyone considering merely pregnancy as such, or planned parenthood. There seems little room for useful comment following the endless tides of discussion reaching an unparalleled ninth wave in the Papal pronouncement. Except, perhaps to point out that although The Pill is still canvassed as the safe and harmless way to birth control, it has not yet been established that it is not injurious to a woman's health. But whatever the chosen method—rhythm, mechanical or oral—it seems clear that family planning is here to stay, not least in the paramount interest of the child.

Even before and beyond chosen parenthood, however, parents need to realize that the pre-natal conditions they provide have a far higher importance than they may have even dimly surmised.

The influence of pre-natal conditions
The long reign of George IV was drawing to a close when a new life was lovingly conceived in the vicarage of Holme, a small village on the remote edge of Dartmoor. The mother-to-be, young, beautiful, gifted and intelligent, decided that this was to be no ordinary child, but a being stirred by the beauties and mysteries of nature, and alive to and in sympathy with all forms of life as well as man. She was convinced that, by the grace of the Master-Builder, it was in her hands to lay the foundations for such a person and to this end she walked on the moor, sketched and pondered, and read great poetry. We may smile at her simplicity and dismiss such pre-Victorian ideas as idle fancies. Yet her son, Charles Kingsley, was to earn a wide reputation as Professor of Modern History at Cambridge, as noble-hearted vicar of a small parish in Hampshire, and as author of many pamphlets on social reform, children's books, novels and poems that are read and loved to this day. Furthermore, there is no doubt in the mind of such advanced medical thinkers in obstetrics as Professor Ashley Montagu that 'what happens between conception and birth

is much more important for our subsequent development than we have till recently realized'.[1]

Vulnerability in the womb
In thirty-eight weeks or thereabouts, the human being grows from a single fertilized cell far smaller than the point of a pin to a creature averaging seven pounds in weight, and a foot and a half in length, consisting of some 200 billion cells of hundreds of differing varieties and functions, all developed from the initial cell. To grow so fast, so much and so variously, is unique in life. None of us can repeat it, however long we live. For this reason the mother, who forms the immediate environment of every individual, has an unequalled opportunity and responsibility to influence her child for its future good or ill during this fantastically crowded period of life before birth.

'I am the tadpole of an archangel,' announced Victor Hugo. Whether or not Everyman becomes an archangel in the end, he certainly resembles a tadpole in the beginning, or rather in the first weeks of existence. Then he begins to shed his tail and develop the nervous system, sex organs and limbs that entitle him to be called a foetus. It is during these first three months, when the cells are developing and differentiating to form organs, that spontaneous abortion is most common and the vulnerability to damage is at its highest. Yet the pregnant woman may be unaware of her pregnant condition until it is so well established that she seeks advice from a doctor or clinic.

Since a firm diagnosis cannot always be made until the twelfth week, when the risen uterus can be felt by the hand in examination, this points to the advantages of early pregnancy testing to establish whether or not conception has occurred, especially where there have been previous miscarriages or it is advisable that habits potentially damaging to the child should be given up.

Vital needs begin with conception
Because things begin to happen to us from the moment of conception, every pre-natal influence is potentially vital from this point onwards. The mother, being the sole source of oxygen, food and shelter, must be protected from any physical or mental harm, for the effects of these will be transmitted to her unborn child in the bloodstream which they share, and she herself must be provided with the best obtainable quality of food and with pure air and water. Again,

oxygen is the primary need. As Professor Ashley Montagu reminds us, 'The most critical single element in the life of a child before birth is his supply of oxygen.'[2] Adults can, and do, fight for this. The unborn, still living in water, cannot. Their blood can only absorb what the placenta provides via the mother.

Preferably not premature

The wanted baby is welcomed whenever it appears but for everyone's sake it is best that it should not jump the gun. Prematurity spells peril. A human being needs to lie snug and protected completing his body systems for the full term of nine months. Born before his time, he will have to cope with the new tasks of breathing, sucking, digesting and eliminating before he is entirely equipped. That means a struggle to stay alive in a new world.

No single pre-natal factor is held responsible for prematurity but there are some important ways of reducing the chance of it. These are: plenty of oxygen (no smoking), no unnecessary medicines, no drugs, and a good diet during pregnancy.

The strongest possible insurance against prematurity with its danger of brain damage, death in the first weeks of life or cerebral palsy is to carry out these recommendations. It is worthwhile considering in full detail how this may be done.

Oxygen for the unborn

Every mother hopes to bear a well-formed infant with the promise of growing up healthy and intelligent. The majority do. But there is far too much physical and emotional ill-health among us twenty or sixty years later for anyone to show complacency about what happens before birth, which can do lasting damage to our mental and physical equipment. A woman may not feel at all concerned about living dangerously herself; but what if this damages the unborn? Every child depends on the quality of what his mother eats, drinks and above all breathes, for his need for oxygen is greater than hers.

The vulnerability of the unborn to a shortage of oxygen is highest in the first three months of pre-natal life and gross malformations due to it occur chiefly during this period. Serious damage to the nervous system and the nerve-sheaths can occur at any time because these continue to develop from the ninth foetal month until two years of age.[3] Where twins are expected, a full supply of oxygen is especially important, for, although there may be twice the amount of blood available, this does not necessarily mean that there is twice the oxygen present and also available.

The importance of oxygen for the pregnant cannot be overrated, since the mother is the only source on which the offspring can draw. The oxygen level in the foetal circulation is only about one-third that of the mother, and there is little margin of safety. It is therefore essential to let nothing interfere with the continuous flow of these minute molecules through the fine hairlike villi of the placenta. For, if the nerve cells are destroyed or the development of blood vessels affected by lack of oxygen, the results will be serious, ranging from cerebral palsy,[4] spina bifida and cleft palate, to the birth marks which are common in prematurity.[5]

It is not easy to obtain a good and steady supply of pure oxygen in any industrial area, where each factory, closely packed domestic chimney and vehicle extracts some of the vital ingredient oxygen, from the atmosphere—as well as polluting it by the addition of a number of harmful elements. Consequently, air which is relatively unpolluted must be sought out deliberately and frequently as in gardens, parks or open country among growing vegetation. Even such an apparently simple matter as nose-breathing can put up your oxygen intake by a critical 10 to 17 per cent over mouth-breathing, whether by day or night. No animal but Man sleeps with an open mouth, and Red Indian mothers were always careful to ensure the habit of nose-breathing by gently pressing together the lips of the papoose in its birch-bark cradle. This is a primitive custom which could well be copied by the sophisticated, with lasting benefit to the child.

Oxygen by vacuum pump
In 1958, Professor Ockert Heynes (Dean of the Medical Faculty, University of Witwatersrand, South Africa), convinced of the great importance of oxygen for the unborn, embarked on an experiment to try to improve the supply, especially during the last weeks of pregnancy, when the placenta stops growing and the heart of the foetus cannot pump blood through it, even though its oxygen demands are greater than the mother is providing. The Decompression or Foetal Oxygenation suit he devised was a sort of vacuum pump in plastic covering placed over the mother's abdomen, and ideally applied for half an hour daily for the last ten weeks and up to the first stage of labour. It was used by him on about ten thousand mothers.

Not one of the babies born to these mothers had cerebral palsy (author's italics), which in Britain is expected to occur in twenty cases out of this number of births, and labour was short and painless for most of the mothers.[6]

Many of the parents concerned were of the opinion that these babies might be extra intelligent compared with others who had not had this treatment and this was apparently confirmed by tests carried out later among the children in Johannesburg. This led to extravagant claims that the 'Birth suit' produced a proportion of brighter babies. However, the results of a subsequent four-year research project of very carefully controlled tests by a Johannesburg psychologist, published in 1968, showed no significant difference in intelligence between a group of babies whose mothers were given decompression, and a control group receiving standard ante-natal physiotherapy alone.[7]

Be that as it may, the fact remains that improving the oxygen supply resulted in *no* cases of cerebral palsy, to underline the primary importance of oxygen for the unborn in every pregnancy.

Factors to be shunned

An old proverb has a timely warning: 'It's an ill bird that fouls its own nest.' Yet how many expectant mothers out of sheer ignorance and lack of thought *do* foul the nest where their child lies. They all need to know that they must look to their habits, and discard those which may be harmful to the unborn. Here smoking stands high on the list.

Smoke knows no sanctions. It has the freedom of the air, and is not content to remain in its place of origin. Every non-smoker becomes a 'passive smoker' in any home or public place where unpolluted air is not ensured by feelings of consideration, or non-smoking notices. However, there is usually some form of ventilation in these places. There is none in the womb, and no escape from the smoke dissolved in the mother's bloodstream. *So every smoking mother is inflicting smoke on her unborn child.* This is now known to have harmful results.

In 1959 the *British Medical Journal* carried a report of a study made in six hospitals in Birmingham of the effects of smoking on the children of about two thousand women. It was found that smoking substantially reduced the growth of the child in the womb.[8] This was a disturbing finding but a far more disturbing relationship between a mother's blood pressure in pregnancy and her smoking emerged from a recent survey by the Head of the Department of Obstetrics and

Gynaecology at Sheffield University. Writing in 1968, Professor C. S. Russell stated that smoking quite certainly reduces the weight of the baby, which may well endanger its life, since he found a death rate of four in a thousand pregnancies where the mothers were smokers.[9] He believes that the harmful effect may be partly due to poisoning by carbon monoxide which is a product of incomplete combustion. This hypothesis is supported by his finding that the surviving babies of the smokers appeared to have a growth leeway to make up. Among the 2200 pregnant women in a wider survey he began some ten years ago, he found that smokers who have had vaginal bleeding in early pregnancy are particularly likely to have premature deliveries between the twenty-eighth and thirty-sixth weeks of pregnancy.[10]

Other substances in tobacco smoke which can pass through the placenta and harm the foetus are nicotine and polonium 210. Nicotine depresses the blood sugar level, increases the pulse rate, and raises the blood pressure, contracting the end blood vessels to the brain so that it receives less oxygen.[11] Polonium 210, which is radioactive, passes into the blood stream attached to the smoke particles and, since it disintegrates slowly, the cumulative effects can be serious for mother and child.[12]

Workers at the University of Freiburg Gynaecological Clinic studied over two thousand pregnancies and reached the conclusion published in 1967 that 'from our investigations and from studying the literature from Japan, Great Britain and the USA and other centres in Germany, cigarette smoking during pregnancy leads to an increase in toxicity, prematurity, abortions and underdevelopment in infants. *Every pregnant woman should be told of the danger and a VETO on smoking pronounced.*'[13]

Some twelve years earlier, it had been demonstrated that mice deficient in a certain factor of vitamin B Complex and certain amino-acids, suffered greater tissue susceptibility to tobacco smoke than those adequately fed,[14] thus emphasizing the great importance of well-based habits of eating when exposure to smoking by others in the household or at work cannot be avoided by mothers-to-be.

Of course, no woman would ever wish to be directly responsible for taking the risk of endangering for life the mental or physical capacity of her child. Yet the evidence above shows that she is doing precisely this when she smokes during pregnancy. It is difficult to understand how ash-trays can be tolerated at any ante-natal clinic. Surely they should be replaced by NO SMOKING notices, coupled with plainly worded warnings to impress on every mother-to-be that smoking during pregnancy can only be regarded as selfish and irresponsible indulgence, which may be bitterly regretted later.

The menace of carbon monoxide for the foetus

Experiments have proved that depriving cells of oxygen can turn them into cancer cells, and malformations and other abnormalities may be induced through the prevention of orderly and normal growth,[15] while certain anaesthetics and analgesics (pain-killers) administered to the mother affect the supply of oxygen to the brain of the foetus.[16] There is a physiological exchange of gases in the human placenta due to the differences in tension of each gas across the placenta membrane.[17] The placenta is a pancake-like structure of cells nourished jointly by both environment and embryo, i.e. by the child and by the parent. It has been called the lungs and liver of the foetus. It is designed to act as a strong-room where the maternal bloodstream stores deposits of food, water and oxygen to be passed on to the growing body as it builds up.

The day may be approaching when small but repeated inhalations by the mother of carbon monoxide, arch robber of oxygen, and the most dangerous of the fumes arising wherever fuel is burned without proper ventilation, may be more widely recognized as having long-reaching and harmful effects on her unborn child. Such inhalations may occur in any average home with any unvented gas appliance, as has been pointed out in Chapter 1, and a case of high blood saturation by carbon monoxide in a foetus *in utero* (a child in the womb) has been medically reported.[18]

NO MEDICINES, *'on tap' or by prescription, during pregnancy*
The thalidomide tragedy opened the eyes of the world to the horrifying effects of an apparently innocent medicine on prescription given to a pregnant woman. In fact, all prescribed medicines without exception can be classified as toxic, to some extent, according to a standard medical textbook, and pregnancy, though an entirely natural condition, is one where a wide variety of substances which may appear to have no harmful effect on the mother, can and do harm her unborn child.

The reason for this extra vulnerability is that the growing cell is far less able than the mature cell to withstand any adverse effect on its environment. In addition, the developing human organism has neither the excretory nor the complicated detoxifying mechanisms, nor yet the equally complex system of enzymes, to deal with any toxins. This explains why the mother may emerge apparently un-scathed from a situation where her unborn child suffers irreparable damage.[19]

All analgesics (pain-relieving medicines) readily penetrate the brain tissues to do their work, and as readily pass the so-called 'placental barrier' to reach the foetus. It is not in fact correct to call this a barrier, since most medical preparations pass through, especially if it is weakened as in cases of diabetes mellitus, low blood pressure or haemorrhage.[20]

The most frequently used of all medicines available to everyone must be aspirin, or one of its fellows, kept in practically every hand-bag, and heaven knows how many masculine pockets. Admittedly it is less toxic than some other preparations for stifling pain while masking the cause. The fact remains that it is known to interfere with digestion, and the ability of the cells to absorb sugar, and to increase the need for oxygen and for every known nutrient. In addition it speeds the loss through the kidneys of calcium and potassium and all the vitamin B complex and vitamin C, extra amounts of which are needed during pregnancy. It should also be clear that if the mother-to-be suffers these losses so, to a far greater extent, does the child she carries. An effective dose for the mother of, say, ten grains, represents about eight times the equivalent dose for the developing child.

A high aspirin intake during pregnancy in rats has been found to produce congenital abnormalities in the litter,[21] while in human mothers it may cause intestinal bleeding and is known to lead to the iron deficiency anaemia from which one in every four woman of child-bearing age suffers![22] It is better to take one or more tablets of vitamin C (100 mg) which overcomes minor stresses causing head-aches and vague pains. If it does not work, here is a warning that the cause lies deeper, and should be put right—not covered up.

Anaemia is usually corrected by the administration of iron com-pounds. Unfortunately some of these preparations not only destroy vitamin E[23] which helps to prevent varicose veins at a time when these are most likely to appear owing to the extra weight to be carried, but they also increase the need for oxygen and are liable to cause liver damage[24] and bring on miscarriages, malformations or prematurity.[25] This is especially so if insufficient protein is eaten, or illness reduces the food intake.[26]

In an attempt to combat the anaemia which is all too common in women in recent years, iron has been added to white bread. But research by Dr P. C. Elwood of Queens University, Belfast, reported in the *Lancet* in 1968, suggests that the type of metallic iron which is employed may be ineffective because it is in a form which is only poorly absorbed.[27] Furthermore, there is another component of today's white bread which is potentially harmful in pregnancy. This is the bleach, chlorine dioxide, which replaced the more harmful agene. Though claimed to be non-toxic, it has the effect of oxidizing essential fatty acids and destroying vitamin E.[28]

Ferrous gluconate is claimed to be the least toxic form of iron[29] but even taking this is quite unnecessary. More than one-third of our daily requirement of iron can be safely derived from wholemeal flour, since this important factor has not been removed in the milling, as in white flour. Merely substituting wholemeal for white flour products of every kind, and eating meat, eggs and plenty of fruit and vegetables, should supply twice the daily amount recommended by the British Medical Association.

Closely rivalling aspirins come the laxatives on which fortunes have been made by those cashing in on what has earned the title of 'The Englishman's Complaint'. These irritate the delicate intestinal membranes, interfere with digestion and absorption of food, and cause weakness of the muscles of the intestinal wall not under our conscious control. The most deplorable laxative is liquid paraffin. Unfortunately this mineral oil is still very widely taken and even prescribed, especially for the pregnant, though its harmful effects have been known for many years. It is not itself absorbed, but hinders the absorption of the fat-soluble vitamins A, D, E and K, as well as carrying them away with calcium and potassium as it is excreted, so depriving the foetus of these essentials. The safest, best and cheapest laxative is ordinary bran (not a breakfast food) costing a few pence at pet shops and corn merchants. It can be stirred into soups, gravy, porridge, etc., or taken with a glass of water before meals. Start with one teaspoon, increasing if necessary to meet the individual need. Although it may cause flatulence at the beginning, this soon wears off, and a regular habit of soft stools is established.

Millions, including many pregnant women, demand 'tranquillizers' because they feel 'nervy' or unable to cope with the effects of their own harmful habits. Such pills can only act as palliatives, and may do a lot of harm if their use is prolonged, as it so often is. They can do nothing to correct the underlying causes. These may be due to fears and anxieties, whether conscious or unconscious, which cause stress and overwork the adrenals so leading to low blood sugar. Or they may be due to low blood sugar caused by the consumption of too much sugar and refined starches which leads to a shortage of calcium, magnesium and vitamin B complex, all essentials for the health of the nervous system. These conditions can best be overcome by simple nutritional improvements.

It has been found that any barbiturate (tranquillizer) given orally collects in the brain, liver, kidneys and spleen of the unborn at a relatively much higher percentage than in the mother,[30] and work with pregnant rats given three commonly used tranquillizers has shown that these resulted in more pre-natal deaths, rendered the off-spring less active and, by depressing the central nervous system, impaired their learning and 'reasoning' ability.[31] So do not ask the doctor for a tranquillizer because you feel tense. Teach yourself to relax instead, for this never produces undesirable side effects and is good for everyone, pregnant or not. It may even be better than a drink and a cigarette for a tense husband too.

Tension and relaxation
Whole books have been devoted to the art of relaxation. Those with the leisure should consult them. Meanwhile here are three simple techniques for relaxing the tense lips and tight mouth in a tight face, constricted ribs, stiff joints and rigid posture arising from physical tension. They are easy to grasp and carry out, and cost nothing but a little time, yet the relief they bring can be great.

1 To loosen up the face and improve the breathing, practise yawning deeply and expanding the chest together. Begin before getting up in the morning. Blow your nose to ensure a clear airway. Lie flat on the back with a pillow under your head, with the legs lying straight down and arms loosely near the sides, palms down. Close your eyes lightly. Now yawn, opening your mouth just as wide as you can, then wider still until your ears crackle, and your nostrils open wide too. At the same time turn your palms slowly upwards, and drawing all the air you can into your expanded rib cage, press your head back against the pillow, and your legs against the bed as you extend your toes as far as you can. Linger over this enormous yawning. Stretch and enjoy it like a cat. Then blow all the air out of your lungs with a long hiss and slowly turn your arms until the

palms face down again, letting your whole body go limp. Now rest your breath. Remember, breathing is a rhythm of three beats, inhale, exhale and rest, and the passive period of rest is the most important for relaxation. Now you are ready for another huge yawn. This time raise your arms as far back as possible above your head as you open your mouth wide, then return them to your sides as you blow out the air. Rest your breath as before. Then repeat from the beginning several times.

These simple movements not only stretch tightened structures. They tone up flabby ones, such as the muscles holding up the head against the pull of gravity, and the diaphragm (separating chest and abdomen) which is not used in shallow breathing. They also improve the oxygen supply and speed up the general circulation of the body, thus helping to relieve tension. Crossing the legs and folding the arms impede all these, and should therefore be avoided.

Loosen bra, suspenders, etc., and do a repeat performance, if you can lie down during the day. If not, sit in an upright chair with bottom and spine supported against the back of it, and legs a little extended in front of the knees, and do it in this position. If performed last thing in bed two or three times, this deep yawning is an excellent preparation for a good night's sleep.

2 Of course, except when yawning, breathing should be through the nose which warms and filters the air. Moreover, an increased volume can be taken in and breathed out if the nostrils are always fully dilated. Practised consciously at first, this can become a beneficial habit, making you ready to move on to complete breathing which includes the abdominal and trunk muscles. With all clothing loosened, lie down on a firm surface with a pillow under the head and the knees drawn up to a right angle. Or sit with the whole back resting against an upright chair. Rest the fingers lightly on the upper abdomen. Breathe out slowly, first from the chest and then from the upper abdomen, until this is well drawn in and sinking against the spine. Pause and rest. Now breathe in, letting the abdomen swell and the lower chest expand fully against your fingers. Repeat from six to twelve times. Gradually you will do this naturally—breathe out, pause, breathe in, at your own rhythm and speed, and you will find yourself becoming more relaxed as you get the habit of full abdominal breathing rather than mere chest breathing.

3 This last technique is directed at all your muscles grouped in a flowing sequence. Strip to bra and pants or loosen all restrictive

clothing. Place a folded blanket on the floor. Lie down on the blanket on the right side, the right leg and foot loosely outstretched in a straight line. Extend the right arm back to lie loosely, palm up, along the back, so that the front of the right shoulder and right cheek are on the blanket. Bend the left arm to a right angle with the body and the left forearm at a right angle at the elbow, fingers loosely extended and palm down. Draw up the left leg to make right angles at hip and knees, and stretch out the right foot. A young child can lie flat on the floor without straining the spine. An adult cannot, having developed the normal lumbar curve. In the position described the whole body is fully supported without strain, whatever the figure. You are ready to begin.

Close your eyes lightly, and breathe in and out in the three-rhythm gently. Now tell yourself that you are going to remind your body by quiet confident commands that it should and can relax each group of muscles in turn until it has given up its unwanted tenseness and lies as limp as a rag doll. Use an even slow rhythm throughout and speak the words inaudibly.

Start with the fingers of the right hand. Say, 'Extend the fingers (pause) and relax.' Suit the action to the words as you say them. However there is no need to move any joint fully. It is sufficient to feel the muscles of extension contract and then let go. Now apply the same command to thumb, wrist, elbow and shoulder. A short pause. Move to the right leg working up from toes, ankle and knee to hip. Apply the same routine to the left arm, then the left leg. You have reached the head. Now say, 'Wrinkle the forehead (pause) and relax.'—'Dilate the nostrils (pause) and relax.'—'Smile widely (pause) and relax.'—'Drop the jaw (pause) and relax', and finally, 'Hiss-s-s-s and relax, hiss-s-s-s and relax, hiss-s-s-s and relax.'

You are now lying completely relaxed in the most restful position possible. Why not perfect these easy techniques by practice?

Better than pep pills

Mothers-to-be complaining of fatigue or exhaustion, which may be due to oxygen deprivation from the inhalation of carbon monoxide or to nutritional deficiencies, tend to ask for prescriptions for pep pills (amphetamines) which, if given, may lead to over-stimulation and habituation if not addiction, leading to a later demand for a tranquillizer. So the vicious circle is set in motion.

In 1968, the BMA warned the Home Office Committee on Drugs

that legislation would be needed if voluntary restriction did not occur.[32] Yet the fact that amphetamines may also be prescribed for slimming purposes when too much weight is put on during pregnancy was disregarded. However, slimming without pills and without hazard can be achieved by the measures detailed in Chapter 10. Furthermore, there is no need to take pep pills for anything. Dried brewer's yeast is a far better booster for personality inadequacies, depression and general morale, without the risk of over-stimulation or addiction. Take one to four teaspoons in a little milk or water with each meal. Reduce the amount if this loosens the bowels too much.

It has been known for many years that certain preparations given for morning sickness increase the effect of barbiturates, depress the central nervous system, inhibit the sympathetic nervous system and cause liver damage.[33] Yet they still appear to be taken for this nausea of pregnancy, in spite of a recent report that they also potentiate (increase) the action of the toxic organophosphates used as insecticides now almost universally present in food, air and water.[34] Any farmer will confirm that he has never seen morning sickness among his pregnant livestock, which are also mammals, but, of course, the grains they are given are whole, with none of the important vitamin B complex removed. Pregnant women could well follow this example by replacing all white flour products by whole meal. Or, if unwilling to take this easy step, they could obtain the missing factors by taking dried brewer's yeast as recommended above to replace any tranquillizer.

One indisputable advantage of The Pill must be that there are now fewer unsuccessful amateur attempts at abortion with such agents as quinine, lead and ergot. A single large dose of quinine has caused a congenital cranial malformation and defective mental development in the infant; lead has been known to cause opacity of the cornea in the infant; and ergot has caused fatal poisoning in the mother.[35]

On the other hand, a report published in 1968 by Dr Richard Doll and Dr M. P. Vessey of the Medical Research Council's Statistical Research Unit has led to a warning that women smoking more than fifteen cigarettes a day should not have prescriptions for The Pill because smoking may accelerate the formation of embolisms which cause thrombosis.[36] Support for this warning comes from the US Public Health Service report that smoking increases the stickiness of some of the minute structures in the blood involved in the formation of a thrombus.[37] For those anxious to take The Pill this is an additional argument in favour of giving up smoking altogether.

Even antacids, given for the heartburn and indigestion which is a common complaint especially around the fifth month, can have adverse effects by 'crowding out' the mineral magnesium which is essential for nervous stability.[38] This complaint can be safely remedied by riboflavin (vitamin B_2) which is an extra need since the baby is now drawing heavily on the mother's reserves and this is 'the choice of the good physician'.[39] It is easily available as part of the vitamin B complex in brewer's yeast taken in a little water with meals.

Antibiotics have become so popular that they are practically insisted on by the ignorant for relatively mild conditions. This means that natural immunity is not acquired, while sensitivity to the particular one prescribed often is, and there has been unnecessary exposure to possible toxic effects. In fact all antibiotics given to the mother are found in the foetal blood, and what may be a therapeutic dose for her may well be lethal for the infant, whose enzyme system is not yet fully developed.[40] Although streptomycin given to the mother has caused congenital deafness in the highly vulnerable unborn child,[41] throat lozenges containing antibiotics were banned by the Food and Drug Administration (USA) in 1966 as being *ineffective* rather than unsafe![42] Commonsense then tells us not to ask for antibiotics, above all when pregnant.

X-rays are now unlikely to be used if a foetus is known to be present, since universal attention has been directed to the dangers. It remains even more important, however, that exposure to radiation should not take place in any case where conception *may* have occurred, in view of the fact that if experienced during the first weeks when only a few cells exist in the embryo, the injury may be fatal. Nor should it be allowed during the next three weeks when the major organs are forming and there is the likelihood of producing gross abnormalities. An expert suggests that a pregnancy test be carried out on every potential mother before any exposure to an X-ray is even considered.[43] If it is even remotely possible that you are pregnant, then ask for this test to be done before you submit to any X-rays.

Soft and hard drugs
Among drugs taken for kicks, for the escape from reality they afford, the non-addictive 'soft' drug LSD has such highly hallucinatory

properties that a young man walked in front of a fast car believing it could not harm him—and was killed. Potential parents who take this so-called mind-expanding drug, or the peyote extolled by Aldous Huxley, may be threatening the physical and mental health of future generations, since it has been shown that considerable damage to the chromosomes of the white cells can be caused, predisposing to leukaemia and other cancers.[44]

Before adjourning its annual meeting in January 1968 the UN Commission on Narcotics repeated its strong warnings on the dangers of LSD, asking for a complete prohibition on the production and use of the drug, and its source materials, except in controlled medical experiments and in established medical uses. A weight of medical evidence was presented of the harmful effects of these so-called lesser drugs. The Commission reiterated the warning that cannabis and cannabis indica, variously known as pot, hemp, dagga, marihuana, hashish, etc., not only distort perceptions of time and space, causing accidents and leading to violence and craving for harder drugs, but can also affect the chromosomes, resulting in serious birth defects and leukaemia among children born to mothers taking it.[45] In some ways LSD can be more perilous than hard drugs, as it is without colour, taste or odour, making it easier to conceal, smuggle and market.

Where mothers have become addicted to the 'hard' drug heroin, their babies may be born with the same addiction. It has been revealed that there were about 800 such babies born in New York City in 1965 who suffered all the agonies of withdrawal in the first few days of life and who often did not survive the ordeal.[46]

Clearly, there is now unmistakable and mounting evidence that practically *every* medical preparation in common use today and every one of the soft and hard drugs is dangerous to the unborn. Especially during that early part of its pre-natal life when the mother-to-be may not even realize that she is indeed pregnant, for the embryo is two weeks old before a menstrual period is missed. The conclusion is obvious: only under the direst necessity and under strict medical supervision should they ever be permitted.

Parenthood means three people
We may eat up to seventy tons of food in a lifetime. Perhaps the most important task of this food is to provide the materials from which a baby is built.

It is a matter for sober reflection that almost every teenager downing 'cokes', over-sweet concoctions and starch, starch all the way, in the fume-laden confines of a café, is destined to become a parent sooner or later. How pitiful that through ignorance or indifference and injudicious habits, a young couple, even if endowed with all the love in the world, can not only besmirch their own well-being but endanger the health and happiness of the child or children on whom all their hopes and fears will later be centred.

Not only does it take three persons to make one parent, but both the parents carry a direct responsibility for the creation and composition of the third person in this eternally recurring triangle. Hydrogenated fats (hardened vegetable oils such as cooking fats and margarine) do not contain the substances necessary for the good functioning of the glands, particularly the pituitary and adrenal. A father or mother-to-be who lives largely on these artificially solidified fats, together with starches, sugars and carbonated drinks, is more likely to become the parent of a defective baby, and, in the case of a mother, to suffer miscarriage.

It was once comfortably believed that the human embryo was even more secure from harm than a bird in an egg. Nutritionists now know that this is not so. It has been clearly learned that the human egg can be, and is, very adversely affected by bad feeding and other habits in either parent. Animal breeders have long been aware that since a new life starts from the conjuction of ova and sperm, it is important that each contributor is in an optimum condition before conception. It is ironical that the valuable germ separated from the wheat grain in milling is *not* put back into the white flour used for feeding humans, but carefully given to stallions and boars.

The effect of food deficiencies on the next and later generations was clearly demonstrated in 1937 by Professor Fred Hale of Texas Agricultural Experimental Station in the case of pigs. He found that curtailment of vitamin A in the rations of either sow or boar, produced abnormalities of eyes, ears and palate. Later he purchased a litter of pigs born blind because a drought in another part of Texas deprived the parents of green food. As long as the rations contained ample vitamin A for both parents, these blind sows produced normal litters in subsequent farrowing. Had a hereditary factor been responsible there would, of course, have been a proportion of blind offspring in spite of the vitamin A.[47]

Working with women who had previously miscarried or borne

defective infants, Dr Evan Shute and the group of physicians with whom he is associated in Canada studied the effect of vitamin E* deficiency in such cases. When the fathers concerned were also given this vitamin prior to the next conception, it was found that out of the subsequent births, the average of abnormal infants fell to only one, where it could have been seventeen.[48]

The need for knowledge of nutritional values
Fortunately many future parents are neither sugar nor 'coke' addicts and they genuinely believe that they are eating well and sensibly. But in point of fact food has become so denatured and devitalized today that it takes a surprising amount of knowledge, awareness, and vigilance to ensure that the choices made cannot either harm the unborn or fail to provide the necessary elements for its optimum development in the womb, and later in the world.

Some forty essential nutrients are required to work together as a team to synthesize the ten thousand or so compounds needed to make and maintain a healthy human body. If these are not adequately supplied the genes and chromosomes, which have an equal need for nutrients, may fail to come up to standard and this may have dire consequences for the future child.

Chronic disease often begins before birth as a result of abnormalities due to abnormal chromosomes. The essential function of the chromosomes is thought to be directing the building of proteins, including the all-important enzymes and co-enzymes. These very complex substances are stimulated by the presence of minerals to behave rather like foremen in charge of the work carried out by the cells.

The cause of the thirty-odd new diseases known as 'congenital errors of metabolism', in which children are born lacking certain vital enzymes, is now believed to be the distressingly inadequate diets eaten by the mothers concerned. For instance, an infant whose liver lacks a certain enzyme, so making him unable to metabolize a substance present in milk and milk products, is most likely to become mentally deficient from an accumulation in the brain of this substance, unless the condition is recognized at the outset. Fortunately, if at once put on a special diet from which this component—dangerous to him but nutritious to the normal infant—has been largely removed, his sanity may be saved.[49]

* One of the fat-soluble vitamins removed by liquid paraffin taken as a laxative, and by the bleach in white flour.

Since an *apparently* sufficient intake of vitamin B complex coupled with high levels in the blood when tested can mislead, experts consider it advisable to increase the intake in all cases where it is likely to be depleted.[50] Depletion may arise from the vomiting of early pregnancy, faulty methods of cooking, excessive consumption of starches and sugars, antacids, baking powder, alcoholism, drinking too many fluids, as well as through taking medicines, drugs, antibiotics, barbiturates, anti-seasick pills and sleeping pills. The latter are often demanded for insomnia which may be due to excessive smoking, the inhalation of domestic fumes, or the taking of pep or slimming pills. A better approach would be to identify and then eliminate these causes, and learn to relax, allowing the return of natural sleep, which is far more beneficial.

Unheeded signposts to danger
Ever since 1910 experimental zoologists have been amassing information about the production of malformation in fish, amphibians, hens, pigs and rats, yet the medical world appeared to remain totally insulated from this highly relevant knowledge. Fifty years later the first International Conference on Congenital Malformations was held in London attended by some five hundred doctors and experts in anatomy, biology, obstetrics and experimental embryology. At this date about 4–5 per cent of babies had abnormalities arising at birth. Then the thalidomide tragedy shocked the world, and the attention of many investigators became focused on such abnormalities.

As long ago as 1918 Dr Sequiera at the London Hospital showed that it was possible to treat with drugs not only an expectant mother with syphilis but also her unborn child. Had the important implications been given the attention they deserved, the birth of millions of stillborn, premature or malformed children might have been prevented. We have been tragically slow to link cause and effect in a passion for pills which has overwhelmed both those who swallow them and those who profit from their manufacture and distribution.

The fact that not every mother taking thalidomide had a malformed baby is of tragic interest especially from the nutritional viewpoint. Why were some stricken and others spared? A possible explanation is that adequate diets provided protection, whereas some of those who suffered may not have been aware of or were indifferent to the need, in pregnancy, not to increase food as such but to eat foods which are nutritionally valuable. This view finds confirmation in some experiments with rats. Where rat mothers had been deprived of certain factors in vitamin B complex during pregnancy, some 60 per cent of their offspring were born with foreshortened limbs, and a lesser percentage of such disabilities also occurred when they lacked other components of B complex as well as vitamin A and vitamin E.[51] Other investigators have found that extremely short and transitory deficiencies of folic acid (part of B complex) during early pregnancy in rats resulted in cleft palates and many other congenital defects,[52] and as long ago as 1939 a survey by the University of Pennsylvania Medical School of the mothers of 154 congenitally deformed children of whom 90 per cent died in the first year showed that 50 per cent of the women had *no milk* and only 1 per cent had one pint weekly, while nearly all of them ate white bread, and very few had fresh fruit and vegetables, resulting in a lack of not only riboflavin (part of B complex) but also of vitamins A, E and C.[53]

Movement and muscles
Not only must a mother-to-be pay heed to what she takes in to her body, she must give thought to how she uses it.

Inactivity means inflexibility and lowered vitality as well as less oxygen absorbed. Therefore too much sitting, whether in a vehicle or gazing at TV or whatever, is not desirable. Taking plenty of exercise, and especially gardening and walking in the freshest air available, increases the amount of oxygen taken in and the tone of the muscles. It is after all muscles, not midwives, that deliver a baby. To have them in good condition, working freely and able to relax at will makes a splendid preparation for the day of delivery and gives confidence in the ability to control the mind and body. All those who are within reach of the ante-natal physiotherapy available at hospitals and welfare centres, are advised to take advantage of their services. These relaxation and exercise classes can be as effective in pregnancy as the much publicized 'decompression' treatment now being tried in over forty NHS hospitals for a variety of ailments such as painful menstruation and backache.

Avoidance of over-fatigue
Lack of oxygen adds another stress to the basic stress of life, reaction to which keeps us alive. This additional stress is resisted by using extra energy which calls for extra cortisone from the adrenals. If this

demand is excessive the adrenals suffer from overstrain, upsetting the general metabolism and probably resulting in a fatty liver. Overstrain of a similar kind can arise from the prolongation of anxiety, emotional stress or excessive fatigue, because these also release an excess of hormones and these latter can pass the placenta to enter the body of the child in quantities that can be harmful. Investigators at the Fels Institute at Yellow Springs have studied the body movements of children before birth and found they were related to the emotional stresses undergone by the mother. During the periods when the mothers were disturbed, the movements increased several hundred per cent. One result of this over-activity is to lower the birth weight, compared to that of a less active child of the same length. He has used up his food in physical activity, so his deposit of body fat is lessened. If a good body weight is wanted, then emotional stability of the mother is desirable and this is adversely affected by fatigue, its surest enemy. Where there are other children and a home to run without help, as well, perhaps, as a job to go to, fatigue becomes an occupational condition. It can be counteracted, to some extent, by the resolve to snatch a few moments to put up the feet, and to avoid over-conscientious spit-and-polish and late hours. The first duty of a mother is to take care of herself, because she carries a child, and other duties should be allowed to slide. In this way she can safeguard against reaching a state of fatigue that a night's rest cannot cure. Indeed the best advice to offer any mother-to-be can be summed up as: 'Say *no* to noxious fumes in the home, smoking, unnecessary medical preparations and all drugs, and the self-robbery detailed in later chapters. Say *yes* to fresh unrefined foods, some of them raw, with sensible exercise, work, relaxation and rest, if you really want to do the best you can for your future child.'

An increasing need for oxygen
As pregnancy advances, the need for oxygen grows not less but more. Dr Grey Walter, the famous brain physiologist, has put this dramatically: 'The convulsive twitching and stretching of the unborn child is evidence that its oxygen supply is lagging behind its needs. With growth the deficit increases, until at the appointed phase of some maternal tide, half suffocated the baby thrashes its way to freedom or disaster.'[54]

While an adequate intake of oxygen is essential for both mother and child throughout pregnancy and labour, the common practice in premature delivery and suspected uterine distress of over-ventilating the mother with room air or supplementary oxygen has been strongly deprecated, since re-analysis of human data and experiments on sheep have shown that this may significantly reduce the oxygen supply to the unborn child and in fact leads to severe asphyxia if prolonged.[55]

Once over the bridge between the world of the womb and the world of air, the infant must breathe or perish. The first breath is the hardest. Thousands of air sacs in the lung have to be expanded from scratch, and this takes about five times the energy required for an ordinary breath. The well-known kitten-like sound at birth is not, contrary to popular belief, a wail of distress. It is an emergency breath, as the hitherto unexpanded lungs (which remain as solid as the liver until expanded) draw in air for the first time after expelling fluid. The move from a watery to an oxygen-laden environment has been safely made when a baby begins to breathe. It is not strictly true to say we breathe because we need oxygen. We breathe because if we did not we should soon begin to need oxygen and should have to either breathe or die. So the cry of the infant announces the onset of the first human hunger, the hunger for oxygen satisfied by the first breath of life. Indeed if the infant fails to cry on delivery, a timely slap elicits this as a reflex action, and life has begun involuntarily.

For the next two or three days breathing is irregular and difficult, for there is the added necessity to clear the air passages of mucus, and here it is that crying is really of value and to be welcomed. Furthermore, the temperature of the room is likely to be below the blood heat (98° F) of the womb, and the poorly focusing eyes must adjust to light after darkness. No wonder there are cries from the newborn as it works at the new business of breathing. This leads on to the conscious control of the involuntary action of breathing which every child must acquire in learning to suck, blow, swallow, cough and especially to speak.[57] Although stress and various emotions may lead to laboured breathing, breathe in oxygen we must, for it is the most automatic and urgent action of a human being. Polluted domestic air thus remains one of our worst enemies from our first breath to our last.

Whether or not they are parents or prospective parents, some women are self-employed, earning a living at home by exercising an art or a skill, or are housewives busy in their homes. There are a number of domestic dangers they may meet while doing their chores, against which a warning is both necessary and overdue.

REFERENCES

1   MONTAGU, ASHLEY. *Life Before Birth* (Longmans, 1964)
2   *Ibid.*
3   BICKNELL, FRANKLIN, MD. *Chemicals in Food and Farm Produce* (Faber, 1960)
4   ROBERTS, DR W. A. B. 'Asst. Gyn. and Obstr. Tutorial', University of Witwatersrand (19 November 1962)
5   TEDESCHI, C. G. *et al. Am. J. Obst. and Gyn.*, 71 (1 January 1956)
6   HEYNES, O. S., MD. *Abdominal Decompression A Monograph.* (Witwatersrand University Press, 1963)
7   LIDDICOAT, RENÉE, MD. *S. Afr. Med. J.* (2 March 1968)
8   LOWE, C. R. *BMJ* (October 1959)
9   RUSSELL, C. S., MD. *Sheff. Univ. Gazette* (January 1968)
10 RUSSELL, C. S., MD. *New Scientist* (9 January 1969)
11 *BMJ* Editorial (4 March 1961)
12 RADFORD, E. P., JR *et al. Science* 143, 247-9 (January 1964)
13 MEY, R. *et al. Univ. of Freiburg Gyn. Ned. Klin.*, 62, 1 (1967)
14 KRESHOVEN, S. J. *Jour. Dental Res.*, 34, 798 (1955)
15 WESTLAKE, AUBREY, MRCS, LRCP. 'Life Threatened' (*Journal of Soil Association*, 8 March 1964)
16 MISRAHY, G. A., MD. *et al. Anaesthes.* (March/April 1963)
17 BARTELS, H., MD. *et al. Am. J. of Obst. and Gyn.*, 84, 1714 (30 December 1962)
18 DREISBACH, R. H., MD. *Handbook of Poisoning*, 4th Edition (Lange Medical Publications, 1963)
19 THOMSON, DR WILLIAM A. R. *New Scientist* (16 August 1962)
20 CABRINI, DENTKOS M. *Am. J. Hp. Pharm.*, Vol. 23 (March 1966)
21 WINNICK, MYRON, MD. *Nursing Outlook*, Vol. 14 (January 1966)
22 KILPATRICK, DR G. S. *The Early Diagnosis of Anaemia* (Office of Health Economics, 1969)
23 WADDELL, J. *et al. J. Biol. Chem.*, 80, 431 (1928)
24 MATTHILL, H. A. *Nut. Rev.*, 10, 225 (1952)
25 VERZAR, F. *Inter Congress Vit. E.* (1955)
26 MATTHILL, H. A. *Nut. Rev.*, 10, 225 (1952)
27 ELWOOD, P. C. *Lancet*, 2, 516 (1968)
28 SHARMAN, I. M. *et al. Brit. J. Nut.*, 14, 85 (1960)
29 THOMPSON, M. M. *et al. Am. J. Clin. Nut.* 8, 80 (1959)
30 MELCHIOR, J. C. *et al. Lancet*, 2, 860 (October 1967)
31 ARMITAGE, S. G. *J. Comp. and Physiol. Psych.*, A45 (2) (1952)
32 *Medical News* (28 November 1968)
33 SAPEIKA, N., BA, MD, PHD. *Actions and Uses of Drugs*, (A. K. Balkema, Cape Town, 1955)
34 FITZHUGH, GARTH O., PHD. *Can. Med. Ass. J.*, Vol. 194, (19 March 1966)
35 *Munch. Med. Wschr.*, 100, 560 (1958)
36 BYRNE, DR ALFRED. *Sunday Times* (29 December 1968)

37   *Ibid.*
38   SHILS, M. E. *Am. J. Clin. Nut.*, 15, 133 (1964)
39   FREDERICKS, CARLTON, MD., BAILEY, HERBERT, PHD. *Food Facts and Falla-cies* (Julian Press, New York, 1965)
40   CABRINI, DENTKOS M. *Am. J. Hp. Pharm.*, Vol. 23 (March 1966)
41   LITTLE, W. A., MD. *Am. J. Nursing*, 66, 6, (1966)
42   *New Scientist* (7 April 1966)
43   RAVENTOS, A. *Am. J. Nursing* (June 1966)
44   HIRSCHHORN, K. *Science*, Vol. 155, 1417 (1967)
45   U.N. COMMISSION ON NARCOTICS. *A.G.M. report* (January 1968)
46   YERBY, ALONSO S., MD., MPH. *New York State Journ. Med.*, 66, 10 (1966)
47   HALE, FRED. *Texas S. J. Med.*, 33, 228 (1937)
48   SHUTE, EVAN, MD. *et al. Vit. E. Symposium Ann.*, New York Ac. Sci. L11, 63 (1949)
49   BICHEL, H. *Bibl. Paediat.*, 81, 63–75 (1963)
50   FREDERICKS, CARLTON, MD., BAILEY, HERBERT, PHD. *Food Facts and Falla-cies* (Julian Press, New York, 1965)
51   MILLER, Z. *et al. Jour. Biol. Chem.*, 237, 968 (1962)
52   MURPHY, D. P. *et al. Am. J. Obst. and Gyn.*, 37, 460 (1939)
53   MONTAGU, ASHLEY, MD. *Life Before Birth* (Longmans, 1964)
54   WALTER, W. GREY. *The Living Brain* (Penguin Books, 1961)
55   MOTOYAMA, E. K., MD. *Lancet* (5 February 1966)

6

Danger. Women at Work

'Out of this nettle danger, we pluck this flower safety.'
HENRY IV PART I

Whether she goes to work or not, a certain part of the housewife's day is spent at work in the home, washing clothes and dishes, cleaning and polishing. The potential hazards of many of the materials she uses are largely unknown and unadvertised, yet ignorance of them can have consequences ranging from the unpleasant to the lethal.

Deodorants, bleaches and cleansers
Few modern housewives make the pomanders or pot pourris that covered up personal and unwanted odours of earlier ages with pleasing scents that could harm no one. Instead, every supermarket and chain store finds a ready sale for agreeably perfumed discs or crystals of para-di-chloro-benzene (PDCB), containing a bleaching agent. PDCB is an insect repellent once used extensively against ants in greenhouses which were killed by the poisonous vapour given off. It is now used extensively as a deodorant. The windows in a lavatory, the smallest room in the house, are generally left open, but in a combined lavatory and bathroom, this is infrequent in winter. Consequently, the continuously released particles of the deodorant weighted by the odour being heavier than air, are trapped in such places and persist indefinitely to be breathed in and absorbed by the skin. The effect on flies, to be seen dead on sills and floors, is obvious. On humans, not obvious but insidiously harmful. In public conveniences, so often situated below ground level, this can do no good to the attendant and can be distinctly unpleasant for visitors.

PDCB belongs to a class of penetrating, persistent and cumulative poisons which can cause widely ranging symptoms such as temporary hoarseness, eye irritation, headache, sinusitis, neuritis, etc., and they can build up to serious trouble whose cause may be totally unsuspected. Perfumed sprays of many kinds have something of the same drawback, for the propellant is of necessity a chlorinated hydrocarbon with the same properties.[1] For all cases of asthma, respiratory and sinus sensitivity they should be absolutely taboo. Incidentally, the nose gets desensitized by the constant assault, so that all that is felt is a stinging in the nostrils, and this may eventually be enjoyed, as sometimes happens with taxidermists who use PDCB, unmasked by perfume, to preserve the skins of birds and animals.

Denture cleansers are generally based on phosphoric acid and sodium perborate which carry a toxicity rating of four: 'very toxic'. They are labelled with a warning to rinse carefully after use, and it is very important to observe this precaution for the latter decomposes to hydrogen peroxide and sodium borate, which is strongly alkaline and irritating.[2] A dentist's tip to use ordinary toilet soap on the brush is a practical and inexpensive substitute, and runs no danger of accidentally poisoning an inquisitive child.

Bleach and lavatory cleansers when combined give off noxious vapours of chlorine gas, and should never be used together. They have caused deaths in the elderly. Nor should bleach ever be mixed with strong rust removers or acids, though it can safely be used with soap, detergents and caustic soda.[3]

Toilet preparations and cosmetics
Talcum powders often contain borax, to which infants are 'sometimes startlingly sensitive',[4] so these should be avoided by any nursing mother as well as anything containing boric acid, such as douches of any kind or mouth washes which might be transmitted through her skin or by contact. In any case, it is undesirable to block many of the pores of the skin through which an infant not only perspires, but breathes, for we all do about a one hundred and sixtieth part of our breathing through our skins.

Removers of lipstick stains may contain per-chloroethylene or trichlor-ethane which are highly toxic.[5] Instead, any washable material should be sponged with cold water, and then rubbed with eucalyptus oil or white vaseline by the finger tips before washing with soap and warm water. The eucalyptus or vaseline should be rubbed on non-washing material, then dabbed with a few drops of ammonia diluted with water, then rinsed well.

Face creams, grease paints and hair dyes may contain lead.[6] This can be stored in the bones without ill effects, but individual susceptibility varies greatly, being increased by fatigue, infections and faulty diet, especially that lacking calcium and vitamin D. Moreover drugs used in some illnesses can release it from store and give rise to poisoning. The symptoms are pallor, frontal headaches, pain in the back and chest with foot and wrist drop which may lead to palsy.[7] An increasing amount is being detected in human blood. This may be partly attributable to the tetraethyl lead in petrol which was introduced in 1923, and gives off fumes of lead when burned in cars. Using this petrol in cigarette lighters, blow lamps or solvents has the additional hazard that when unburned it contains fat-soluble organo-lead compounds which can be absorbed if spilt on the skin,[8] and great care should be taken to avoid this. Since few modern cars run on the old-fashioned petrol without lead, this may be difficult to obtain, but would obviate this danger.

The Royal Society for the Prevention of Accidents (RoSPA) stresses that the greatest care must be taken when using a hair lacquer spray not to smoke, not to use it near any heating appliance, to store out of direct sunlight and to keep even empty containers out of reach of children, for there will still be vapour in an empty container. The hydrocarbon used as the propellant carries the added peril that it is highly inflammable—hence this stringent warning. The explosion that will occur if an empty container is heated is staggering, and a hair spray if set alight will hurl a roaring jet of flame over two feet and turn a head of hair into a ball of fire in a second.

Do-it-yourself dry cleaning
Per-chloroethylene and tri-chloroethylene are present in most liquids sold for dry cleaning by the amateur but their safety is very much in question. The Federal Government Division of Occupational Health in the USA set up a study programme with a ten point list of 'urgent problems' which included the factual dangers of tri-chloro-ethylene, and carbon-tetra-chloride.[9] Early in 1970 it was announced that the use of carbon-tetra-chloride in household cleaners was to be banned by the FDA (Food and Drug Administration) since it had been found so extremely hazardous that warning labels were not enough to protect the public.

Carbon-tetra-chloride has been outlawed in Great Britain by many suppliers of household dry cleaning fluids since the national press in 1966 drew attention to a report by the American National Safety

Council listing a widespread number of deaths in America of people succumbing to the sweetish fumes. Although tri-chloroethylene was referred to in this report as thirty-five times less toxic, there have evidently been second thoughts about this also. Stain removers containing the much more seriously toxic carbon-tetra-chloride are, however, still marketed in this country, following the Home Office view that no action is necessary to ban them, since they all carry warning labels. Nevertheless, these are usually in such small print as to be overlooked by the user and, in any case, none of them carries any warning of the danger arising from using them after drinking alcohol or if smoking. These have been found to add so considerably to the danger of injury to liver and kidneys that they are banned in the USA. Nor do the labels point out that susceptibility of reaction is also increased in anyone with a calcium deficiency, poor nutrition or a malfunctioning liver.

Launderettes for dry cleaning

Now that launderettes have mushroomed in every town or village, and provide additional facilities for dry cleaning, the hazards from these sources have grown enormously. The agent used, per-chloro-ethylene, is definitely classified as a toxic solvent and there must be good ventilation whenever it is used.[10] Industrial safety rules in the USA limit the permitted concentration of its vapour to 200 parts per million by volume. This vapour is three times heavier than air, having a molecular weight of ninety-five, with the mean molecular weight of air approximately twenty-nine, hence the heaviness of the fumes and the fact that they concentrate at a low level. So, although the obligatory ventilating shaft inside the machine comes into action when the doors are opened to take out the cleaned garments, the vapour from the solvent builds up a concentration low down by the door where the client is standing. This makes it especially serious for small children who accompany their mother and may be holding on to her skirts as she operates the machine and removes the garments.

In commercially run businesses it is the practice to hang all finished garments or other material in a draught for twelve hours so that the fumes may all be removed before the work is returned to the customer. In the do-it-yourself process the customer extracts the load, puts it in the boot or on the seat of his or her car and drives home. Unless the articles have been *sealed* in a plastic bag, this is highly unsafe since the fumes which continue to be given off may cause the driver to turn giddy or even become unconscious. (Note that per-chloro-ethylene is used in hospitals for its anaesthetic properties.) Who wants to run the risk of being rendered unconscious while driving? But there is no trace of a warning about the possibility of this effect if precautions are not taken to avoid it.

When requested by the local Medical Officer of Health (who had received complaints from users) to put up a notice in his establishment drawing attention to these dangers, one owner recently refused point blank, saying it would make his customers reluctant to use the machine. An MOH has no power, at present, to compel anyone to comply with his request for at least a warning notice of the dangers, nor to insist on better ventilation other than that provided by a swing door which only opens to admit customers, and a fan (which indeed is seldom working) in the cramped and overcrowded room in which the machines are available. It is to be hoped that no fatality will occur before this power of enforcement is awarded him by law. If it should be your lot to be present when someone becomes drowsy from these fumes, the procedure is to remove the sufferer, lay him down in the open air and call a doctor at once

Since the National Association of Launderette Owners believe that there is room for expansion beyond the 4000–5000 already in use, we may assume a similar surge upwards in the number of dry-cleaning machines sharing these premises. It has been pointed out that although these may be money-spinners, they remain a risk investment. They certainly constitute a risk in more dangerous directions. There are amateur owners who seem quite unaware that they are handling a fluid with fumes that may be damaging not only to their customers but also to themselves as they remove the used product.* Anyone unfortunate enough to have such a machine installed under their living premises may also suffer dire consequences. For example, Mrs J. writes, 'We have been in a maisonette for fifteen years above the shopping parade here, and have been happy and in our usual robust health until the cleaners were installed in the empty shop below. In all our thirty-eight years of married life, my husband has never had a day off for ill health, but during the last nine months has been really ill and on two occasions had to be

* Owners of launderettes who must regularly remove and replace the cleaning fluid should provide themselves with special oxygen supplying apparatus.

away and mostly in bed, suffering from what the hospital term bronchial asthma, due in the beginning to a virus on the trachea and sensitivity in the lungs.' The Corporation, the firm supplying the chemical and the MOH have proposed modifications to the plant, but in the meantime Mrs J. and her husband have chosen to find other accommodation. As trapping sunbeams presents less difficulty than preventing the percolation of fumes through ordinary ceilings and floor boards, they have surely acted wisely. But what of future tenants? How long before they find themselves similarly afflicted? Will they have the knowledge to know what is affecting them?

Stain removers

Among household stain removers sold for special purposes, those for tar, rust and soiled furs may contain xylene, toluene and ortho-chloro-benzene, which gives them a toxicity rating of four, equal to that of carbon-tetra-chloride, long discarded by many manufacturers for this reason. Xylene and toluene are toxic by all portals of entry, and although absorption by the skin is too slow to produce systemic poisoning, it can result in a characteristic dermatitis attributed to the removal of the protective layers of the skin.[11] The symptoms caused by inhalation resemble those of carbon-tetra-chloride.

Tar, bicycle oil and crude oil picked up on beaches can all be quite safely removed with eucalyptus oil. On a pad of material, with blotting paper underneath, the eucalyptus should be worked into the stain using some cotton wool with a gentle rubbing movement until the stain disappears. Rust on metal surfaces should be dabbed with paraffin, or soaked in it for several hours, then dried and rubbed with an emery cloth until it is all removed. The cleaning of a typewriter, except by the skilful and careful use of an old tooth brush or a pin to clean the letters, is best left to an expert.

Soap

Soap has been in use as a cleaning agent since prehistoric times and specimens discovered in the remains of a soap factory in the ruins of Pompeii show that then, as now, it was made of alkalis combined with acids of oils and fats. This combination is a menace to dirt and undesirable bacteria but to nothing else, and it is noteworthy that even in this detergent-ridden era, surgeons still scrub up with soap before an operation. Furthermore, soap residues present no disposal problems, being easily broken down by the bacteria in sewage systems and the soil. In fact soap can look back on a long and wholly blameless past. Not so detergents.

Damage by detergents
The history of synthetic detergents goes back only a few decades, but is increasingly stained by indictments of far-reaching damage to human beings, wild life, and the environment, locally and generally, since they ousted soap as a cleaning agent.

The chemists who manipulated molecules to make the first synthetic detergents, unfortunately failed to foresee the effects of dumping what now amounts, in Great Britain, to some thousands of tons of residues of the surface-active and other materials of which they are composed into waste disposal systems every year. This has created serious difficulties wherever it occurs, which today means universally.

Synthetic detergents have been in use for about forty years but were at first restricted to the wool industry where they were used to remove fat from the fibres. Then they were made into shampoos to take the oil out of human hair. This they do most successfully. It remains questionable how good it is, in the long run, to have one's hair left dry and brittle, and the skin of the scalp so denuded of its natural and nourishing oils that it is liable to shed its outer layer in dandruff.

The use of plain white soap followed by a rinse with one tablespoon of cider vinegar in half a basin of warm water to remove any possible trace of soap scum, has no such drawbacks.

Soap rationing brought detergents into our homes and these became a profitable new industry which succeeded in very largely replacing soap. This raised vast new problems for those concerned with waste disposal, and when it was found that a glass of drinking water might show a head of froth like beer, research began in earnest. Only then was it realized that these much vaunted cleaning agents had many disadvantages. Many of the first users landed themselves in hospital casualty departments with serious and persistent fungus infection of the nails. The original treatment—the continuous application of gentian violet—was so unsightly and slow that research was undertaken. This produced a preparation made from another species of fungus which proved more satisfactory. Meanwhile the manufacturers, alerted to possible drawbacks, sent round bands of young women in uniform to warn households to wear gloves to protect the hands and not to use their product so generously.

In 1956 a report by the Ministry of Housing and Local Government[13] showed that domestic detergents were polluting domestic water supplies, and that the concentration of detergent in British rivers ranged from 0·2 to 4·9 ppm. While conceding that the surface agents and foam themselves are not highly toxic to animals when fed to them for several years, the Committee expressed the opinion that 'the possible occurrence of serious effects over a much longer term cannot be ignored . . . and the possibility will need to be kept under careful review'.

It was estimated in 1960 that in dry weather we might be drinking as much as three milligrams daily in tap water to which must be added about another two milligrams taken in food and drink, often prepared in utensils washed with detergents and not carefully enough rinsed.[14]

Percolating filters, activated sludges, sewage works and healthy rivers work hard through their saprophytic bacteria (scavengers on decayed and decaying materials) to break down the organic wastes they receive. The phosphates and surface-active agents in the wastes of synthetic detergents now present in all these places provide them with an excessive food supply and this leads to over-population. There follows a lack of oxygen, since they have consumed it all, and a repression of the re-aeration of the oxygen depleted waters. This leads to the replacement of these useful aerobic organisms by their evil smelling and putrefying anaerobic brethren which mingle with algae, sewage fungi and colonies of bacteria, etc., to starve the water of light and air, seriously affecting plankton and the fish which feed on it.[15]

Although we have gradually followed the USA example of replacing the so-called 'hard' detergents which are resistant to biological breakdown, by 'soft' ones which are more readily degradable, it is considered by experts that there is no decrease at all in the amount of material still to be dealt with, because we are buying more detergents.[16]

Although it has now been removed, the completely inessential foam, added to detergents in the past merely to pander to the housewives' traditional belief in its virtue, was for years an unmitigated curse smothering sewage works and workers in faeces-infected clouds, or towering over their heads to be blown over the countryside or float along waterways killing water weeds and fish.

Enzyme additives
The incorporation of enzymes in certain brands of detergents available in this country has succeeded in raising them to top place among the many on the British market. They have proved harmful for users as well as workers and are now arousing concern and enquiry.

Laundries have used enzyme solutions to remove such resistant stains as egg yolk, gravy and blood for over fifty years. It is only recently that they have invaded the domestic market with much blowing of trumpets, thanks to clever packaging and promotion, and the ageless lure, for the uninitiated, of the magical.

In reality, enzyme action is a biological fact and has nothing to do with magic, although those who have suffered from its action might feel that it may have some connection with the machinations of black magic. We live in a world of enzymes and could not indeed live without them. They are plant or animal proteins acting as catalysts or foremen who direct the action of water on other proteins, and they play an important and continuous part in the processes of any cell which allow it to feed, function and reproduce. Certain stains resist removal from materials because the proteins they contain act as binding agents, and the commercial enzymes added to detergents work powerfully at the job of speeding the process of removal.

However, tests by the Consumers Association have shown that, abracadabra apart, there was little effective difference between expensive enzymatic or cheap 'standard' detergents providing overnight soaking to loosen stains was employed with the latter. Except the difference in price, of course. Too often this leads to the erroneous idea that a dearer buy means a superior product. On the contrary, grave disadvantages from their use have recently come to light and should be more widely known.

Damage by enzymes to users, workers and materials
While the makers claim that enzymes do not attack live cells, a leading skin specialist disagrees, and considers that they can attack the skin's protective layer of dead cells, inflame the live tissue underneath and leave the skin more vulnerable to other potential irritants in the detergent. He says he has seen many cases of eczema of the hands attributable to these causes. A more recent report from the Department of Dermatology, Hallamshire Hospital, Sheffield, points out that a number of patients suffering from unusually severe dermatitis of the hands had all used an enzymatic detergent shortly

before, had no previous history of eczema or any other relevant skin disease, and had not been affected by using a 'standard' detergent. In the majority of cases there was in addition to the acute eczema a secondary eczema due to photosensitization (sensitivity to light) on distant parts of the body. Patch tests had established the enzyme additives as the causative irritant, and suggested that the eczema caused would be a particularly serious and virulent type.[17] Among the women employed as home helps in Nottingham, twelve developed dermatitis after using enzyme detergents, an incidence of 5 per cent.[18]

Damage to the skin should not be regarded lightly since the skin is the first line of defence against bacterial invasion, but there is a far more serious risk in the breathing in of enzyme dust. This is difficult to avoid in using, or worse still in making, such powders. There have been medical warnings that the resultant damage to the surface cells and the covering of mucus which protects the lungs and its appendages could have grave consequences.[19]

When the manufacture began of Aerial (with Radiant one of the most popular brands of enzyme powders) it was found that several workers in the Newcastle-on-Tyne factory suffered from asthma or flu-like symptoms from breathing the air laden with enzymes, and a similar effect has been reported from the USA. As a result of a survey carried out by Professor Richard Schilling of London University new and strict control measures have been enforced in detergent production by the makers in Britain.

Enzymes are sealed off, special ventilation provided and special medical checks applied to would-be employees. However, it is still only in these factories that the health hazards have been investigated, and so far nothing appears to have been done either to inform or protect the user.

It is clear from the published figures [20] that there has been a steady rise in the sale of detergents in the United Kingdom in the last seven years, the figure for the past year standing at some 260,000 tons, of which some 38,000 tons has gone down our own drains, the rest being exported. It is surely time to call a halt to this personal pollution of our environment. The way is simple enough in all conscience and could cause no possible harm but only good to every form of life. We can all of us, in our homes at least, return to the safe use of soap or soap flakes which have none of the disadvantages of detergents.

Hints on the use of soap flakes and soap
So-called 'hard' water contains calciums, magnesium and iron compounds which combine with the fatty acid of soap to form an insoluble scum instead of a good lather. Such water should be softened when hot before adding the soap flakes by the addition of one dessertspoon of powdered borax per gallon of water.

Before washing, obstinate stains such as blood and fruit juices should be soaked in one pint of warm water with one tablespoon of liquid ammonia for three to four minutes and then removed and well rinsed.

Coloured fabrics should always be submitted to a preliminary test in some inconspicuous place and if the colour is affected should be neutralized at once by sponging with a weak solution of white vinegar and water then well rinsed and washed.

Stains of the black oil found on beaches, tar and bicycle oils, can all be removed by the eucalyptus oil we associate with colds in the head. This will not hurt the most delicate fabric, it is entirely safe for user and fabric, and leaves no unpleasant odour. Put a pad under the stain and using cotton wool work the oil well into the wrong side, then rub gently, repeating until the offending mark disappears.

Washing up with soap flakes presents no problem if a few drops of cloudy ammonia are added to the water. Every housewife should follow the excellent lead given by Dade County, Florida, USA, with a population of about one million, including the City of Miami, which in 1963 banned the sale or use of detergents in its whole area. No hardship need be entailed in giving up these damaging cleaning agents.

There is indeed only one purpose where detergents are preferable to soap in the household. Flame-resistant fabrics can have the finish impaired by soap powders, but are unaffected by detergents.[21]

It is becoming increasingly difficult to buy a frying pan which has not been coated by a silicone to make it non-stick. This contains an aliphatic or aromatic solvent which turns into a toxic vapour if the contents of the pan burn. Who among us has not had this happen sometimes to the breakfast bacon? The toxicity rating is from three to four which makes this a hazard to be avoided.[22] Though stainless steel and copper-bottomed pans are dear, and good enamel and iron are scarce, they are worth saving up or searching for. Cheap enamel is not to be recommended in combination with any acid, and enamel jugs should never be used for home-made lemonade, as antimony may be dissolved out and result in poisoning.[23]

Don'ts for home decorators
The Institute of Practitioners in Advertising estimated that in 1962 there were over eighteen million do-it-yourself enthusiasts in Great Britain, of whom over eight million were women. Only a fraction of these seem aware of the perils concealed in the wares they use so blithely, in spite of warnings by the manufacturers and others.

Paint strippers, lacquers and removers may often contain inflammable additives and also xylene, already listed above as hazardous. If absorbed through the skin, these are toxic and liable to cause a transient euphoria, followed by headaches and giddiness leading to confusion and ultimate coma.[24] The body should always be kept well covered while working, and all exposed areas of skin washed after spraying, nor should they ever be used indoors unless good ventilation can be ensured. It is far safer to use a blow-lamp though this should not be run on the usual car petrol because the anti-knock content gives off lead fumes when burning. In fact, the Post Office has a rigid rule against this, and issues a special petrol for telephone repair jobs.

Paint itself can be perilous today. The polychlorinated biphenyls used in recent years in paints, resins and plastics are toxic and 'they are in fact regarded as an industrial hazard and threshold limits for them in air have been advised'.[25] Nor is this all. Some paint manufacturers have incorporated insecticides in their wares and this causes untoward effects in numbers of people. However, paints are still available without additives.

Shopping
Inevitably every woman goes shopping for domestic goods. How many of us are careful to look for the BEAB mark (safety specification to British Standards) when buying such electrical appliances as washing machines, irons, hairdryers, electric blankets and so on, or cots, prams and other nursery equipment? Yet these standards have been devised and awarded to protect us and our households from the possible dangers of goods not conforming to these safety standards. They should be much better known and demanded by every shopper.

Fire risks in homes

Fires in industry cause the heaviest financial loss, fires in homes the heaviest loss in lives. The major causes of household fires are well recognized. They involve faulty electrical wiring and apparatuses, the use of oil, gas, coal and wood, smoking, and children playing with matches. Preventive measures against them entail no overloading of electrical circuits, attention to wiring, no extension cords where they can be worn by friction, adequate fire guards, care in the kitchen and with ash and cigarette ends, and no matches left in reach of children.

Largely unrecognized causes of fires in the home are the aerosols, of which an estimated 221 million were sold in 1968 in Britain, polystyrene tiles, cleaning agents, TV sets, and plastic outfits for children. Aerosols, now dispensing anything from deodorants to paints, are dangerous because they may contain an inflammable content like hair lacquer or a liquid propellant like butane gas. These can explode when heated, even by exposure to direct sunlight, because they are pressurized. Even when empty they still contain vapour and must never be thrown on a fire for disposal. Of course, every aerosol carries a warning to keep away from warmth but only too often these warnings have been disregarded.

Home decorators have been repeatedly warned that they are risking life and property when they employ the cheapest standard polystyrene tiles for walls and ceilings since these are inflammable. They continue to buy about twenty times as many of these as the self-extinguishing type which stop burning when the flame is taken away but sell at about twice the price. So far no action has been taken by the Home Office, but the Royal Society for the Prevention of Accidents has expressed its concern at the rising sales of these potential fire-raisers.

Owing to the risk of causing fire, petrol, naphtha or benzene should never be used indoors as cleaning agents, nor should petrol ever be stored indoors. When mixed with air this may form a vapour which can be ignited by a pilot light on a gas cooker or any other flame.[26]

Television sets can overheat and burst into flames if the ventilation holes provided at the back, are not left free so they should never be shut in a cabinet when in use for some time, or pushed against a wall.

It has been claimed that four-fifths of fatal burnings are due to clothing catching alight.[27] This spotlights the usefulness of Children's Nightdress Regulations (1964) and questions the advisability of allowing children to wear play outfits made of plastic, which is so easily combustible. The existing tests for fire risks in clothing materials are clearly not sufficient for the many new man-made fabrics constantly reaching the markets, and it was good news to hear that British Standards Institution Textile Division was trying to produce a new safety standard.

A minor point about hearthside fires of any kind is the undesirability of sitting for long periods with bare or stockinged legs extended in front of the fire-place. This is responsible for the mottled skins seen in so many elderly hospital patients, especially those with poor circulation, who are most liable to do this because their feet are generally cold. The effect is due to the infra-red rays emitted which, with wave lengths of 12,000–7700 Angstrom Units, have the power to penetrate deeply into the skin, causing a breakdown of the iron in the red blood cells, and it can lead to secondary anaemia.[28]

Preventing accidental poisoning of children
It is estimated by the Royal Society for the Prevention of Accidents that every week in Britain hundreds of children, mostly under five, are killed or have to undergo medical treatment because we do not keep household poisons out of their reach. There are three simple ways in which parents could prevent these unnecessary tragedies:

1 NO household cleaners, bleaches, disinfectants, paraffin, polishes, etc., should be kept under the kitchen sink. Pots and pans can be stored here safely but these potential killers cannot. All these dangerous substances should be stored on a high shelf or cupboard out of reach of small children and when in use should never be transferred to soft drink bottles, cups or glasses.

2 NO medicines should be left about. Any still in use should be kept in a safety medicine cabinet which is either kept locked or operates with a closing device which needs two hands to open it. Any old medicines should be flushed down the lavatory pan.

3 ALL garden poisons such as sprays and insecticides, etc., should be under lock and key.

N.B. Even cosmetics are safest in a locked drawer of the dressing table as far as inquisitive little fingers are concerned, since for any infant, toddler or young child the natural place to put anything is the mouth.

Hazards in the garden
Old-fashioned tools thrown down in the garden with the business

side uppermost are a familiar danger in the garden and one that can easily be prevented by a little thought and commonsense. A newer and more lethal hazard is provided by the rotary mower, increasingly popular in this country. Figures from the USA, where its use is almost universal today, show that the horrific blade, whirling at 4000 rpm, can slice off a hand as if it were a dandelion, causing some 75,000 amputations and other wounds every year. Important suggestions to ensure safety in use are as follows:

1 Always wear leather shoes which offer some protection. Never go barefoot or wear canvas shoes when using the machine.
2 Before using, rake away every single one of the smallest obstacles, such as nails, bits of wire, or stick, since these can be hurled like bullets by the blade.
3 Avoid going near roots of trees, stones, or bricks.
4 Stop the motor and make sure the blade has also stopped before clearing the discharge shute.
5 NEVER allow anyone, and least of all any child, anywhere near.

A Sussex vicar was recently unlucky enough to lop the ends off two fingers, and not long after, damage five of his toes while using a rotary cutter.[29] One of his parishioners commented as follows:

> *There was a vicar near Rye*
> *Whose parishioners said with a sigh,*
> *His sermons are splendid,*
> *The church well attended,*
> *But his grass cutting makes us all cry.'*

Bonfires should always be cut to a minimum since they are a source of smoke carrying CO and cancer producing benzepyrenes which can stream in through any open door or window even in a smokeless zone.

If a bonfire is unavoidable, never throw on any discarded battery from a torch or radio or an aerosol container, even if empty. These will explode and may cause serious accidents, and the batteries could spread a toxic mercury vapour.

All the hazards referred to can best be avoided by making better choices of materials, or using them more sensibly. It is up to us to make the choice—danger or safety.

REFERENCES

1   GLEASON, M. N. *et al. Clinical Toxicology of Commercial Products* (Balton Williams and Wilkins, 1963)
2   *Ibid.*
3   *Ibid.*
4   BICKNELL, FRANKLIN. *Chemicals in Food and Farm Produce* (Faber, 1960)
5   GLEASON, M. N. *et al. Clinical Toxicology of Commercial Products* (Balton Williams and Wilkins, 1963)
6   SAPEIKA, N. *Actions and Uses of Drugs* (Balkema, Cape Town, 1955)
7   GRAY, C. H. (Editor) *Laboratory Handbook of Toxic Agents* (Royal Institute of Chemistry, London, 1966)
8   HILLS, J. B. G., BSC. Personal Communication (1 December 1967)
9   *Safety and Rescue,* Journal of RoSPA (January 1967)
10   *The McGraw Encyclopedia of Science and Technology,* Vol. 12, 146
11   GLEASON, M. N. *et al. Clinical Toxicology of Commercial Products* (Balton Williams and Wilkins, 1963)
12   DAVIS, DOROTHY V. 2nd Edition, *New Domestic Encyclopedia* (Faber, 1967)
13   *Report of the Committee on Synthetic Detergents* (HMSO, 1956)
14   BICKNELL, FRANKLIN *Chemicals in Food and Farm Produce* (Faber, 1960)
15   KLEIN, L. *River Pollution,* Vol. II, 'Causes and Effects' (Butterworths, 1962)
16   *Board of Trade Business Monitor* (IIIrd Quarter, 1969)
17   JENSON, N. E. *BMJ* (31 January 1970)
18   DUCKSBURY, C. F. J. *et al. BMJ* (28 February 1970)
19   STUART-HARRIS, C. H. *Science Journal* (January 1970)
20   *Board of Trade Business Monitor* (IIIrd Quarter, 1969)
21   LOW, LIA. *Keep it Clean* (Bodley Head, 1967)
22   GLEASON, M. N. *et al. Clinical Toxicology of Commercial Products* (Balton Williams and Wilkins, 1963)
23   BICKNELL, FRANKLIN. *Chemicals in Food and Farm Produce* (Faber, 1960)
24   GLEASON, M. N. *et al. Clinical Toxicology of Commercial Products* (Balton Williams and Wilkins, 1963)
25   *Nature,* Vol. 16, 226 (January 1968)
26   CARPER, JEAN and GUNDRY, ELIZABETH. *Stay Alive* (MacGibbon & Kee, 1967)
27   *Ibid.*
28   CLAYTON, E. C. *Actinotherapy and Diathermy* (Balliere Tindall, 1941)
29   CARPER, JEAN and GUNDRY, ELIZABETH. *Stay Alive* (MacGibbon & Kee, 1967)

7

Insecticides Indoors

'Nobody knows how many cases of illness result from masked effects of chlorinated hydrocarbons.'

JOHN HILLABY

For many centuries women have attacked their traditional foes in the home—flies, fleas, wasps, bugs, beetles, cockroaches and moths. If not always completely effective, traditional weapons have never recoiled on the user. Now we have changed all that. Since the advent of DDT in 1939 with its hundreds of followers among the man-made molecules known as the chlorinated hydrocarbons (or organo-chlorines), not only are there more insects breeding strains resistant to all insecticides but humans are realizing that they may be harming themselves. Insects can chemically change the molecule of an insecticide to an innocuous substance. Man cannot.

In 1961 the late Rachel Carson drew the attention of the world to the insidious dangers inherent in the extensive use of these powerful, penetrating and cumulative poisons. Reaching us as residues in food and drink through all the links in the food chain, and through our immediate environment, they have the capacity to destroy our guardian enzymes, block our energy-producing processes, and begin those changes in certain cells which we call cancer.

F. E. Egler's impassioned statement of the case against injudicious control of pests by these synthetic insecticides in an issue of the publication *Bio-Science* met with storms of protest, not least from those financially involved. He wrote, 'The problem of pesticides in the human environment is 95 per cent a problem, not in scientific knowledge of pesticides, not in scientific knowledge of environment, but in scientific knowledge of human behaviour. In the affluent society whose god is the income per share, the profit motive is paramount.'[1]

There has been no lack of reassuring anti-alarmists. Typically, they conclude that a state of storage in human fat is reached with a continued intake of these chemicals, that this concentration will not increase and that experiments with rats and dogs have shown no harmful effects, although it is admitted that 2·5 ppm of DDT, aldrin or dieldrin has an effect on reproduction in mammals, causing an increase in pre-weaning mortality among the offspring.[2] Such statements overlook some highly relevant reports giving a totally different picture, as follows:

1 Every man has his own poison equation, his own particular constitution, which in the last analysis determines the effect a poison will have on him.[3]

2 Autopsies on 271 patients dying in hospital showed that those who had used DDT extensively *in their homes* (author's italics) had levels in their tissues three to four times as high as those using a minimum, one case having 50 ppm of DDE, a metabolite of DDT, in the liver fat. The investigators were impressed by the great variability in individuals, and commented that if food had been the primary source, there would have been little variation.[4]

3 Experiments with rats showed that the DDT concentrations in the brain increased during ten days of partial starvation and that this concentration was as high following many small doses as after one large one. Furthermore, debilitated rats died at levels of DDT less than half that killing healthy rats.[5]

4 Other rat experiments have shown that amounts of only 5 ppm in the diet produce alteration of the cells of the liver leading to necrosis (disintegration)[6] and that levels of 3 ppm in the diet of rats inhibits an important enzyme in heart muscle.[7]

5 Tests on seventy-five people in the USA with no occupational exposure to DDT showed levels of DDT ranging from zero to 34 ppm, but averaging 5·3 ppm.[8]

6 In Somerset in 1967 samples of body fat from 101 persons showed an average of only 2·35 ppm of DDT, but one male had none, one female of eighty-seven had 12 ppm and two other females aged sixty-nine had 15 ppm each.[9]

7 A controlled study with humans inhaling very small amounts of DDT showed that although only a few molecules reached the nasal passages to be carried directly to the brain, there were brain disturbances, including one or all of the following symptoms—dimness of vision, headache, inability to recall words or concentrate on a topic, loss of balance, difficulty in swallowing

and a stuffy or dripping nose, with some evidence of a cumulative effect from successive exposures.[10]
Experimenters use healthy young humans, or animals that have been
specially bred and carefully fed and looked after. How can these be
compared with a random sample of the people who fill surgeries and
hospitals because they are not healthy? Yet those are the people
exposed to and using these insecticides in their homes.

According to a Russian paper appearing in 1968, some fifteen
hundred cases of DDT poisoning have been established, including
those reported by Morton Biskind and many others. But the report
concluded that the true incidence has not been revealed because it has
been so largely unrecognized and incorrectly diagnosed on account
of the non-specificity of the symptoms which may include gastro-
enteritis and nausea, vomiting, gastric pain and diarrhoea, headache,
running nose, cough, sore throat, joint pains, muscle pains and
polyneuritis, symptoms which persist for months despite treatment.[11]

Many have tried to dismiss Rachel Carson's *Silent Spring* as
'Science Fiction written with a magic pen', or worse. Nevertheless,
within nine years of first publication its warnings have been justified
and its aims, to some extent, achieved. Sweden banned all DDT and
related insecticides for a test period of two years from 1 January
1970. Denmark banned DDT, aldrin, dieldrin and lindane on the
grounds that they are 'dangerous to animal and plant life and in the
long term to human health' as from 1 November 1969. Norway
banned them from the same date. Canada restricted the use of DDT
by 90 per cent from 1 January 1970. Australia has announced the
rapid phasing out of DDT on farms. DDT has been banned in
Michigan and Arizona and partially in California. The National
Audubon Society has announced a national campaign to prohibit
the use of this insecticide anywhere in America, stating that DDT has
'calamitous effects on nature, and, we think, indirectly on man'.
But Britain still hesitates, although it has been reported that the
Government's Advisory Committee on Pesticides is in favour of
curbing their use. Why wait for a government lead? We can ban them
for ourselves today and change over to the safer alternatives available.

DDT in aerosols and powders against flies and fleas
In what form does any housewife buy DDT, and where? Usually as
an aerosol. Nothing is simpler. She walks into any supermarket,

grocer's or chemist's shop and picks up some pleasant looking container, easy to squeeze, which releases an invisible cloud of particles to settle on the floor and other surfaces and kill flies and wasps. Most of these contain some pyrethrum (a natural product of plant origin) for its quick knock-down effect. Unfortunately this is rarely the only ingredient, probably for reasons of economy as, at present, pyrethrum flowers for making the powder must be hand-picked. Somewhere on the container the small print may read DDT, lindane or dichlorvos. How many ever look for this? There may be even less adequate labelling, and certainly no indication that these are chemical poisons with a cumulative effect on human beings.

Lindane in vaporizers and paints as insect killer
Ever since the Food Hygiene Regulations came into force as part of the Food and Drugs Act in June 1956, laying the responsibility for keeping food free of fly-borne infections firmly on the shopkeeper, electric vaporizers of lindane have spread like the plague not only in shops but in hospitals, schools, canteens, etc., and even in homes. Yet shops depending solely on meticulous cleanliness and open-front refrigeration still maintain equally high standards without vaporizers or danger, and are still to be found. The comment of one such storekeeper when asked why he had not followed the current fashion seems worthy of record. 'What would any of my customers think if they saw a fly drop dead over my bacon? They'd think there was something wrong with my bacon!' They would not be far wrong. What makes such vaporizers so undesirable?

The American Medical Association through its Council on Pharmacy and Chemistry waged a two-year campaign against the use of lindane vaporizers, and in 1954 published a report containing a grave warning on the dangers involved.[12] It stated that 'single doses given orally to experimental animals have been reported to be moderately toxic, whereas inhalation of vapours and fumes is highly toxic . . . Recently, it has been discovered that lindane is stored in significant amounts in the brain and functioning liver tissue of certain species of laboratory animals and that in relatively high doses it may produce profound and long-lasting effects on the central nervous system.'

In his *Handbook of Poisoning*, published in 1963, the Professor of Pharmacology at Stanford University School of Medicine, California, stated, 'Electric or other vaporizers should never be used in living quarters, or *where food is stored, prepared or served.*' (Author's italics.) He also advised that organo-chlorine or phosphate insecticides should not be applied where *body contact with residues is likely to occur.* (Author's italics.)[13]

In 1968 a report in the *Quarterly Bulletin* of the Association of Food and Drug Officials pointed out that when lindane was used in thermal vaporizers 'protection of foods and surfaces is not achieved by covering or packaging with common wrapping *except for metal*', (author's italics) and that the rate of its disappearance from contaminated substances was not constant or uniform.[14] According to another investigator, tests revealed that in a room where no lindane had been used for nine months, and eight windows had been left open at intervals for a total of one and a half months, samples of flour left for five weeks picked up 3·6 ppm of *lindane emitted from the furniture and fabric.* (Author's italics.) The conclusion drawn being that contamination of food is not necessarily avoided if vaporizers are used daily for short periods when food stores are empty.[15]

This lindane is the dangerous substance dispensed by electric vaporizers used on the advice of the suppliers 'overnight when the room is unoccupied and closed', for the effectiveness does not lie in the production of insecticide in the air but in the re-crystallization of the insecticide *on all surfaces* [author's italics] in the room. Thereafter a fly landing on such a surface is killed.' Even the Ministry of Agriculture, Fisheries and Food, in its recommendations for the protection of operators using gamma BHC (lindane is 99 per cent gamma BHC) advises washing hands before meals and after use. How to keep hands uncontaminated when every surface in the room is spread with an invisible re-crystallization of the chemical is anybody's guess. As for small children, with their habit of licking any and every surface, it is a sobering warning that there is evidence that, weight for weight, lindane may be one hundred times more toxic for men than for mice.[16]

Besides occurring in aerosols and vaporizers, lindane is now incorporated in many plastic emulsion paints. These contain what is described as an insect control additive (IFCA), in plain words 0·14 per cent lindane, also known as gamma BHC. It is claimed to kill 'all flies, moths and all known insects which settle on the painted surface', and when tested by the Consumers Association and reported in *Which?* in 1965 was found to be very effective. A letter in the correspondence columns of the *Observer* (7 August 1966) from a reader who was unable to sit even for a few minutes in a room he had had painted with one of these paints, drew many letters from others who had suffered similarly. However, as there are still available equally excellent paints free of such noxious additives, these alone should be used.

The safe alternative is to use only a pure concentrate of pyrethrum. An even cheaper and better method is to hang a fly paper in the kitchen and have a fly swatter elsewhere in the home. (For lavatory use see Chapter 7.) As for fleas, Flit, that old acquaintance of all who have lived in Africa or travelled abroad, has had DDT and lindane added to the original pyrethrum powder, and Keatings powder, once made of pyrethrum only, has gone the same way. They are best avoided. Vacuum cleaning daily, mopping stone, lino or wood floors with paraffin, and using pure pyrethrum should be effective deterrents, under British conditions at least.

Organo-phosphates
Malathion for pests on plants and pets
Among the second major group of insecticides are the organo-phosphorus compounds, which include malathion. The regulations issued by the Ministry of Agriculture, Fisheries and Food stipulate that malathion should not be used if 'under medical advice not to work with organophorus compounds'. How many gardeners consult their doctors before spraying their roses, or other plants? How many housewives read the regulations before using it, as advertised among the sundries in seedmen's catalogues, on their pets?

The public has often been assured that malathion breaks down rapidly and is not stored in the body as are the organochlorines. This is so, but there is one highly important proviso. The liver must be functioning normally for this to be carried out. There are many drugs, conditions and insecticides damaging the liver, and if the liver enzyme responsible for their breaking down has been destroyed, the full force of the poison is felt, and the toxicity rating is high.[17] Furthermore, malathion has been found to prolong the sleeping effect of barbiturates considerably[18] and if repeatedly exposed, individuals may be sensitized to subsequent exposure, damaging the circulatory system. Insecticides which are safe both for pet and owner can be obtained, and so can leaflets with detailed advice on control of pests in the garden without resort to organo-chlorine or organo-phosphate compounds. (*See Useful Addresses, pages 122–3*)

DDVP (*Dichlorvos*)

Another organo-phosphate, sharing the capacity of malathion to inhibit human cholinesterase activity and so interfere with the transmission of nerve impulses, is dichlorphos known as DDVP. This is recommended for homes and kitchens, as well as for every other imaginable building, by the firm making the thermostatically controlled electrical volatilizer which disperses it in the air. These units are installed on a yearly rental basis which includes a maintenance service and one year's supply of the insecticide in solid form and packed in special refill cups. The maker claims that 'the effect is cumulative, so that within a few days all surfaces become toxic to every type of insect pest'. How toxic they may become to young humans we have yet to discover.

When employed as an impregnation on polyvinyl chloride, DDVP is sold equally freely as Vapona strips by another firm. They are used extensively and increasingly throughout Europe, in South Africa, the USA and Australia, not only on farms and where food is consumed, but in homes and even on dog collars. According to the makers' instructions, 'it is made in such a way that it breathes out minute quantities of insecticide into the room. And goes on doing so for as long as three months non-stop!'

Although carrying the approval of WHO and UK Pesticide Safety Precautions Scheme, the safety of these strips was questioned in October 1969 by Professor Goran Lofroth of Stockholm University in a paper read at the Children's Cancer Research Foundation Meeting in Boston, USA. Basing his doubts on recently published and unpublished studies he suggested that these DDVP emitting strips have potentially serious effects on healthy adults when used precisely according to instructions, exposing the household to substantially more than the safety level recommended by the World Health Organization.*

The *New Scientist* editorial commented, 'That serious doubt has not already been cast on the safety of DDVP is at least partly due to the practice of the manufacturers of submitting unpublished papers to bodies responsible for evaluating pesticides.' (Unpublished and therefore uncriticized.)

Pet lovers should note that veterinary workers have observed

---

* One strip is meant to be hung per 1000 cubic feet. Yet it is recommended for use 'in small rooms such as kitchenettes and toilets'. How many of these, averaging some 7 ft by 7 ft by 10 ft reach even half that cubic content?

severe dermatitis among the side-effects of DDVP dog collars, and the more serious failure of dogs exposed to DDVP to respond to anaesthesia, as well as death from minimal doses of barbiturates.[19] This has obvious implications for humans who may need an operation urgently, or take barbiturates for any condition.

Measures against moths

Moths and men have been enemies probably as long as men have worn wool, and DDT was in fact discovered by a Swiss chemist looking for a mothproofing agent for fabrics. But DDT has for years been superseded for this purpose by a related compound, dieldrin, which is about forty times more toxic when absorbed in solution through the skin.[20] It can be stored in the fatty tissues of the body, so that long after exposure it can give rise to fits simulating epilepsy, in any period of physiological stress.[21] Yet few people are aware that they and their children may be in daily bodily contact with it throughout the winter and often into the summer.

Here is a part of its history:

Dieldrin only came into general use in 1950 when it was widely used to replace DDT, mosquitoes having become resistant to DDT. Soon it became one of the most extensively used of outdoor insecticides in spite of the terrible destruction of wildlife that followed, not to mention the many cases of poisoning among spraymen, reported among others by Wayland Hayes in 1959 in the bulletin of WHO, based on his lengthy investigations in Africa, the East and Far East.[22] It was also found to be so persistent that residues were present in soils nine years after application, in potatoes when used against wireworm, and in the fat of sheep slaughtered soon after its use for dipping.[23] In 1962 it was banned in Britain for seed dressing of spring cereals mostly because of bird and animal casualties. Its general use was restricted in 1964, and it was banned for sheep dipping in 1965–6. The remaining uses were 'under active review in 1969'.

Many of those primarily concerned with ecology have pointed complacently to these wider horizons of the environment from which dieldrin has been exiled. They have failed to point to the highly relevant fact of where it is still to be found as a refugee from justice: in the closest environment of all—in contact with our human bodies. How does this occur?

Today in Britain as well as in many other countries, most woollens and a proportion of other textiles—except for baby yarns, 'for certain reasons'[24]—are treated with dieldrin at levels of up to 200–300 ppm to make them mothproof and it is also added to dry-cleaning liquids for the same purpose.[25] Yet one looks in vain for a label to this effect, except infrequently on men's suits. Has there been a conspiracy of silence on this subject? Consider the macabre facts.

In 1959 a special investigator had reported that dieldrin is a toxic substance which is freely absorbed by the skin; that any given dosage is absorbed more readily by a large area of skin; and that bathing the entire body daily with soap and water is essential when contact is over.[26] Admittedly, this was a report on men spraying the chemical. The same criteria surely apply to all those wearing this substance in contact with their skin, in view of the report of a scientific investigator in 1961 that dieldrin is dissolved out by human sweat and the soluate absorbed by the skin[27] and the statement by an expert, in *The Clinical Toxicology of Commercial Products*, published in 1963, that dieldrin is readily absorbed by the skin, resulting in systemic poisoning, *without skin irritation* (author's italics).[28]

Furthermore, in November 1967 a report from the County Analyst of Somerset on organo-chlorine insecticide residues in human fat, noted that the mean level of dieldrin for Somerset was no less than in the 1964 survey, when it should have been lower following the ban that year.[29] He seems to have been unaware that the wearing of mothproofed textiles could account for this anomaly.

Most serious of all, dieldrin is one of the carcinogens, and according to cancer expert W. C. Hueper, there may be special dangers for the young, since the younger the animal exposed, the surer the production of cancer.[30]

Perhaps the most fitting comment is that of Professor Goran Lofroth, 'Treatment of textiles and fibres with dieldrin seems to be an effective way to expose man to this highly toxic and carcinogenic compound.'[31]

Safe alternatives for home storage of woollens
Knowing the needs of any creature is a help in combating its ravages. Recall some facts about the private life of the clothes moth. Losing water as it breathes through the pores and spiracles, in its skin, it must absorb water direct from damp or dampish air. So although modern central heating with its warm houses shortens its life cycle and

increases the number of generations, the drier indoor air is a threat to its continued existence. Again, it prefers material soiled by sweat, excrement or spilled food, which appear to provide certain minerals, vitamins and proteins. So brushing well, airing in the sun, and putting away nothing that is not scrupulously clean, remain as effective protection as in the days of Elizabeth I.

Should you wish to make doubly sure without the use of the organo-chlorine sprays proffered by the chemist's counters, ask for naphtha moth balls.* However, you are most likely to be offered discs or balls only resembling these, but containing PDCB which is in fact one of these same compounds and is to be avoided. In fact, old-fashioned mothballs are scarce since oil-based gas plants replaced the old-fashioned gasworks making gas from coal, which produced the naphthalene (not an organo-chlorine) from which genuine moth balls are made. However, there are other effective repellents. Among these are cedar shavings placed among stored fabrics, or according to Mrs Beeton a strip of linen moistened with genuine turpentine and laid in drawers, wardrobes or chests for a single day three times yearly.

If unlucky enough to get moth infestation in any fabric of the pre-mothproofing era, soak a piece of cotton material in hot water, lay it over the fabric and press with a very hot iron until the cloth is dry, in order to destroy any unhatched eggs.

Ants, cockroaches and wasps in the house
Traditionally, ants were destroyed by preparations based on arsenic, well-known as a favourite means of murder from the Borgias onwards. It is still employed against that invader of South African homes, the Argentine ant. These are not a problem in their own land, where nuptial flights mean heavy slaughter by birds. In their new habitat, with a changed habit of staying underground for the ceremony, these have multiplied into a menace, which the British are fortunate to be spared. All ants are tough, however, and they have survived even DDT and DDVP. The recommended bait of the Ministry of Agriculture, Fisheries and Food contains 1 per cent trichlorphon, which is an organo-chlorine and therefore undesirable.

---

* If you have been lucky enough to buy some naphtha balls to store away baby clothes, be sure to wash the clothes thoroughly before use, as naphthalene has been known to cause acute anaemia in the newborn.[33]

Safe alternatives

A mixture of equal parts of borax and icing sugar (which acts as the lure) thoroughly amalgamated in a bowl with a pestle or wooden spoon so that they do not separate is far cheaper and entirely safe. It can be used as a powder, or diluted with a little water and poured down and around holes or points of entry into the house, or other places frequented by ants, who carry it away to the nest where it does its job by upsetting their boron balance. Since the amount of boron required for health by plants and animals is in the region of one part per million the margin of excess for an ant is minimal, and there can be no danger to soil or other animals. It is essential to keep the mixture in a tin clearly labelled 'Poison' and locked away except when taken out for use, as it could cause illness in a child or someone who mistook it for plain icing sugar. Used as a powder, this is also very effective as a bait for cockroaches and has the same advantages.

Wasps can so easily be lured by jam, fruit or stale beer, that trapping should always replace poisoning. A jar containing any of these with enough soapy water to make them sink to the bottom and drown, so keeping the surface free for newcomers, can be placed outside windows to waylay any would-be visitor. Any that elude the trap can be swatted like flies.

It has been found that the effect on the liver of any toxic agent (which includes all the chemical insecticides) is increased if alcohol is taken regularly.[32] Taken compulsively, as in chronic alcoholism, it has other and incalculable ill effects.

REFERENCES

1 EGLER, F. E. Bio-Science, 14 (11 November 1964)
2 VAN RAALTE, H.G.S., MD. Ind. Med. and Surgery, 24 (Shell International Research, The Hague, 2 February 1965)
3 SCHENK, GUSTAV. The Book of Poisons (Weidenfeld & Nicolson, 1956)
4 RADOMSKI, J. L. et al. Food and Cosmetics Toxicology, 6 (21), 209–20 (Pergamon Press, 1966)
5 DALE, W. E. et al. Science, 142, 3598 (13 December 1963)
6 LAUG, E. P. et al. Jour. of Phar. and Exp. Therap., 98, 268 (1950)
7 ORTEGA, P. et al. A.M.A. Arch. Path., Vol. 64, 614, 22 (1957)
8 LAUG, E. P. et al. Jour. of Phar. and Exp. Therap., 98, 268 (1950)
9 CASSIDY, W. E. et al. Month Bull. Min. H. and Pub. Health Lab. Service, Somerset, 20, 2–6 (1967)

10 KAILIN, E. W., MD. *et al. Med. Annals Dis. Columbia*, Vol. 35, No. 10 (October 1966)
11 POLCHENKO, V. I. *Gigiena i Sanitariya*, 33 (March 1968)
12 COUNCIL ON PHARMACY AND CHEMISTRY, *J.A.M.A.*, Vol. 156, No. 6 (1954)
13 DREISBACH, DR R. H. *Handbook of Poisoning*, 4th Edition (Lange Medical Publications, 1963)
14 LINDGREN, D. L. *et al. Residues Review*, Vol. 21 (Springer Verlag, 1968)
15 DYLE, C. E. *Food Trade Review*, 33–5 (1963)
16 HAYES, W. J. *Proc. Royal Society.*, B. 167, 101–27 (1967)
17 MURPHY, S. E. *et al. Proc. Soc. Exp. Biol. and Med.*, 100, 482–7 (1959)
18 ROSENBERG, P. *et al. Prox. Exp. Bio. and Med.*, 98, 650–2 (1958)
19 SMITH, J. *Am. Vet. Med. Ass.*, 153 (12 June 1964)
20 COMMITTEE ON TOXICOLOGY *Jour. Am. Med. Assoc.*, Vol. 172, 2077–80 (April 1960)
21 LURIE, J. B. *Letter in BMJ* (13 March 1965)
22 HAYES, WAYLAND J. *Bull. WHO*, 20, 891–912 (1959)
23 WILLEMSE, A. G. S. *et al. Science.* Vol. 143, 682 (28 February 1964)
24 Letter from Patons and Baldwins Ltd., Scotland (1 August 1969)
25 LOFROTH, GORAN PROF. *New Scientist* (5 December 1968)
26 HAYES, WAYLAND J. *Bull. WHO*, 20, 891–912 (1959)
27 MAIER BODE, H. *Med. Exp.*, 5, 68–72 (1961)
28 GLEASON, M. N. *et al. Clinical Toxicology of Commercial Products* (Balton Williams & Wilkins, 1963)
29 PEDEN, J. D., FRIC. *et al. Monthly Bull. of the Min. of H. and Pub. Lab. Service*, Somerset, Vol. 26 (November 1967)
30 HUEPER, W. C. 'Environmental and Occupational Cancer', *Public Health Reports Supplement* 209 (National Cancer Institute, 1948)
31 From original MSS partly reproduced in *New Scientist* (5 December 1968) (By courtesy of Professor Goran Lofroth)
32 SAPEIKA, N. *Actions and Uses of Drugs*, Dept. of Pharm. Univ. of Cape Town (Balkema, 1955)

USEFUL ADDRESSES

A. 1 AEROSOLS consisting of pyrethrum and free of organo-chlorines or organo-phosphates are manufactured by Messrs Cooper, McDougal & Robertson, Ltd, Berkhamsted, Herts. and The Py Co. Ltd, London Road, Great Shelford, Cambridge.

   2 HOUSEHOLD SPRAYS consisting of capsules of pure pyrethrum concentrate complete with sprayer are manufactured by The Py Co. Ltd, London Road, Great Shelford, Cambridge.

   3 UNITS using ultra-violet light, and reminiscent of a lantern, killing flying insects indoors are manufactured by Rentokil Laboratories Ltd, 16 Dover Street, London, WIX 4DJ. They can be purchased or rented.

B. 1 HONEY FLY CATCHERS manufactured in Ireland are distributed in the UK by Kay Brothers, Hurst Street, Reddish, Stockport, England.

   2 DUSTING POWDER called Herbisect for cats and dogs containing no organo-chlorides or organo-phosphates can be obtained from Henry Doubleday Research Association, 20 Convent Lane, Bocking, Braintree, Essex.

C.   A BOOKLET entitled *In Place of Poisons* is obtainable free from Henry Doubleday Research Association, 20 Convent Lane, Bocking, Braintree, Essex, on receipt of SAE.

D.   THE PUBLIC may get advice by telephoning the undermentioned Poison Centres in an emergency:

     LEEDS 30715
     NEWCASTLE 25131
     BRISTOL 32041 (Ext. 138)

8

Alcoholism—Hidden Danger to Health and Happiness

'I am distressed for thee, my brother.'

2 SAMUEL 1.26

Ever since the unrecorded date of the first fermented drink, alcohol has played a part in man's intimate life history deserving not only interest but enquiry. No need to enumerate the delights. But what of the dangers? What are they? Who are involved? What are the effects? How can these best be tackled, and by whom?

The progressive disease of alcoholism
The use of alcohol, clearly, does not make an alcoholic, or few of us would escape the label. It is only the abuse of alcohol which causes the progressive disease of alcoholism which is now on the increase in many countries of the West, including Britain. It is indeed only during the last thirty years that alcoholism has been officially and medically accepted as a disease, because the abuse of alcohol has been found to change for the worse the nature and function of our body cells with corresponding effects on our moods and mental capacities. When this happens, there is an apparently irresistible craving for alcohol, the very compound that caused the change, and addiction to alcohol and the disease of alcoholism has begun. This addiction makes an alcoholic, and once an alcoholic, always an alcoholic.

A world authority on the subject has described alcoholism as the biggest public health problem in the world. Such a problem in no way diminishes the moral involvement but places it squarely on us all. Not only on the alcoholic and on his family, but on all of us in the society in which we live. Most definitely this is not an anti-social complaint to be concealed by subterfuge and mistaken loyalty, but an illness to be brought into the daylight so that it may be treated and deprived of its deadly powers to destroy the unhappy victim and the health and happiness of his closest relationships. For although alcoholism is a cruelly destructive, complex, chronic and progressive illness that can lead to utter degradation of body, mind and spirit, it can be arrested and held in check. It is imperative though, that the attack on it falls on the disease and not on the patient, however low he may have sunk in his misery, for he is a very ill person. The civilized and humane do not deliberately scourge the sick, nor pour laughter or scorn on open wounds.

Who are the alcoholics?
In 1961, Dr E. M. Jellinek, consultant for Alcoholism to the World Health Organization, in his book *The Disease Concept of Alcoholism*[1] differentiated five types, with symptoms depending on custom, culture and region, but these seem to be relatively unimportant variations to the large question of what defines an alcoholic. The clearest definition for the layman appears to be that given by a highly educated alcoholic (whose disease was eventually arrested) and confirmed by the National Council for Alcoholism of the USA. There may be heavy drinking but not alcoholism, for alcoholism depends on 'Not whether it is controllable, but whether it is controlled'. The dividing line occurs because the alcoholic is powerless and cannot control alcohol, and in consequence his life has passed out of his own management.

The term alcoholic conjures up to many people a dirty dead-beat, a down-and-out at the back door, but only about 5 per cent can be so described in this country today. We have left behind the gin-sodden lower strata of the Age of Reason and the navvies of the Brunel era responding to the gin shops' invitation to get 'Drunk for 1d.' or 'Dead drunk for 2d'. The alcoholics of the Atomic Age more nearly resemble those of the nineteenth century with its prime ministers, squires and parsons under the table together, to whom we have now added well-paid teenagers and well-to-do women. It has been pointed out that as a result of increased spending power an increasing number of teenagers are developing into alcoholics in their twenties.[2] Furthermore, in a recent survey carried out by two leading psychiatrists, it was found that one half of Britain's women alcoholics belong to the upper social circles, compared with a quarter of the men, though the total ratio of male to female in another survey was estimated to be about four to one.[3]

It is mostly the affluent who can afford to be alcoholics today, yet many are quite ordinary worthy people in all spheres of life, who either do not recognize that they suffer from alcoholism, or conceal the fact because of the unfortunate stigma still attached to it. This constitutes one of its greatest dangers, for being a progressive disease the longer alcoholism is left untreated, the more serious the effects and the probability of a fatal ending if the course is not checked, as can be done by cutting out alcohol for life.

Why does anyone become an alcoholic? No one has yet produced a clear-cut and indisputable answer. There appear to be two main factors—the influence of social attitudes to over-indulgence in alcohol, and a craving for it which may be physiological and/or psychological.

Influence of social attitudes

In primitive cultures and societies, drinking and even drunkenness is a group affair. There is a pattern of festivities where these take place without incurring censure, but apart from these planned and organized orgies there is little drunkenness and no alcoholism. Western society has no such safety valve, and nations differ widely in their attitudes and consequent behaviour, with its influence on national patterns of drinking.

Vineyards in Spain were a legacy from the retreating Moors, who as good Moslems ate grapes and raisins, but drank no wine. For a Spaniard, however poor his home and conditions, wine is the invariable accompaniment of a meal but no glamour is attached to it any more than to bread, and no belief that to drink it is a sign of good fellowship. This unromantic attitude coupled with the sense of dignity and self-respect that is innate in the peasant as well as the grandee, may be largely responsible for the lack of drunkenness and alcoholic problems in the country as a whole.

France, with the highest alcoholic rate in the world, causing the death of one person in every twenty-six minutes, has for many years suffered from a situation arousing deep concern among her doctors and statesmen.[4] In 1960 a lead in a safer direction was given by the then Prime Minister, M. Mendès-France, whose milk-drinking habit was widely publicized, with the establishment of milk bars to encourage the idea that milk is a drink for adults as well as the young, a long-accepted custom in Spain and Spanish America. Today only a labelled bottle may appear on a poster, and it is even forbidden to show liquor being poured or held up to the light for admiration, so strong is the concern and the attempt to take the glamour out of alcohol. But it remains an intractable problem for a number of reasons, which, fortunately for Britons, do not apply in this country.

It has been said that the French are literally supported by alcohol. One out of three voters depends on the production and sale of it for a living; wine is regarded as indispensable; large quantities are drunk throughout the day—an average of three litres (over two pints) being considered quite usual and proper for a working man, who may spend one fourth to one third of his monthly wage on alcoholic beverages;[5] and 85 per cent of school-age children drink cider, beer or diluted wine as a social habit. Not surprisingly, there is widespread chronic poisoning by alcohol, though rarely overtly disturbed behaviour.

As for the financial losses, Professor Robert Debré, whose son was French Foreign Minister, said in Paris in 1968 that alcoholism cost his country at least £58 million annually, from immediately related diseases such as cirrhosis, with another £200,000 for road accidents, and some £6 million for accidents at work.

Although Italy has more land under vineyards than France, there is a far lower consumption of alcohol. Intense social disapproval of drinking during working hours, and the habit of drinking only with meals and in the family circle, where more than one litre daily is regarded as excessive, means there is little scope for drunkenness or dependence, and alcoholism is rare.

An expert in alcoholism visiting South Africa in 1960 drew attention to the fact that he found drunkenness there not only tolerated but considered amusing, an attitude which could only be deplored as childish and immature. Where glamorous advertising on every hoarding was aimed at giving a social cachet and sexual significance to drinking at any time, it was only to be expected that the percentage of alcoholics of about one in every fifteen was said to rank with that of the USA which comes second after France in its figures.

Alcoholism in the USA involving millions of alcoholics has for long constituted a very grave public health problem. It has been attributed to the oscillating attitude of either strict condemnation or frank vicarious admiration, skilfully stimulated by the acknowledged masters of Admass appeal in advertising. None the less, general concern about alcoholism and the measures taken to reduce and contain it are much higher than in Britain, or possibly any other country, and we are all indebted to the USA for the great conception of Alcoholics Anonymous, which began there and spread round the world.

A survey in 1970 by a research team at George Washington University in Washington DC estimated that out of a population of 201 million there may be nine million alcoholics in America, about one-third more than a government estimate of a few months earlier. The report urges that every medical student be given comprehensive training in the diagnosis and treatment of the disease.

The pattern in Britain somewhat resembles that of the USA. Wine is replaced largely by beer and spirits, and these are not drunk continuously during the day or with meals, but as a rule after working hours or the evening meal. This produces a sudden rise in the level of alcohol in the body, which, if excessive, leads to drunkenness. In England drinking takes place mostly in public houses which aim at providing a pleasant social atmosphere. In Scotland on the other hand, where little effort is made to provide any comfort in public houses, and women are discouraged, pathological drinking is more frequent. Mere drinking shops appear to lead to more drinking.[6]

Perhaps the most revealing light on the potent effect of social attitudes is thrown by the figures relating to the Jewish population of New York State who contribute only 1 per cent of all white first admissions with alcoholic psychoses to state mental hospitals. This has been explained as due to lack of taboos on restrained social drinking, but very stern disapproval of excess, linked with the fact that personal conflicts do not appear to be expressed in indulgence, but find some outlet in moderate drinking.[7]

A craving that can kill
Medical opinion is divided as to whether any physiological or other organic deficiencies exist as pre-disposing factors. Dr Roger J. Williams announced to the American Medical Society in 1957, when he was President of the Society and Director of the University's Biochemical Institute, that he believed a biochemical basis for alcoholic craving had been discovered by scientists working on the problem. There appeared to be a large amount of evidence that in alcoholics the appetite-regulating centre of the brain became malnourished, and as a result easily poisoned by alcohol or its metabolic products. Experiments with animals had shown that deficiencies of

vitamin B complex could cause them to drink alcohol steadily. Methods too had been worked out for detecting potential alcoholics in childhood, and it was hoped that by adjusting the faulty diet such individuals could be saved from becoming victims of the disease. Later work by Dr Williams and his co-workers showed that rats were more ready to drink alcohol when the supply of sugar to the brain was reduced, and they sought to confirm this finding by pointing out that diabetics with high blood sugar are rarely also alcoholics.[8]

On the other hand, evidence that deficiency of iodine influences the free choice of alcohol in place of water by rats, whose preference for alcohol fell when the lacking iodine was added to the diet, has since been submitted by workers at the State Research Laboratory at Helsinki.[9] Some investigators have claimed that alcoholics in hospital given two-hourly meals rich in protein, were no longer alcoholics. Others again have pointed out that rat reactions to alcohol when lacking certain amino acids suggest that the medical treatment of alcoholics should pay attention to the protein as well as the vitamin content of the diet.[10] More recent writers, however, dismiss the evidence for any physiological or other deficiency and state baldly that 'craving has not been shown to occur before drinking has taken place'.[11]

Nor has the psychological aspect been overlooked, and maladjustment to life stresses first encountered in childhood has been blamed for the neurosis which has preceded compulsive drinking.[12] Other experiments on humans have shown that alcoholics eating too little and drinking too much, a combination very commonly encountered, can produce in themselves an abnormally low blood sugar which can end in unconsciousness followed by death.[13]

However, whichever comes first, the craving or the uncontrolled drinking, the grim fact of alcoholism remains: it is a psychosomatic disease responsible for an enormous number of cases of suffering and death.

Some effects of alcoholism
The dangerous effects of alcoholism on the body and personality extend increasingly and harmfully into domestic, social and economic spheres. The severity of the symptoms and physical effects depend on the strength and amount of alcohol consumed, though generally following a somewhat similar course. This begins by irritating the lining of the mouth, and a theory that this may lead to cancer of the

mouth is being investigated by doctors in Brooklyn, according to Dr James Kimmey of the USA Public Health Service. The irritation extends down the gullet to the stomach and upper part of the intestines, causing nausea, distention and lack of appetite leading to gastritis. If drinking stops, so do these symptoms.[14] If it does not, lack of appetite, from the high caloric but non-existent food value of the alcohol,* results in severe malnutrition. A vicious circle, leading to an impaired liver, has been set in motion. However, if drinking stops this can be checked, but if it continues the usual progress is to cirrhosis, which kills about 50 per cent of its victims.[15]

Other symptoms occur, predominantly in the nervous system which cannot use proteins or fats to replace the block in its supply of energy from carbohydrates, owing to deficiencies of vitamin B complex, especially B_1. This gives rise to a particularly painful neuritis of the extremities which must have treatment in bed by adequate diet and supplementary vitamins.[16] A recent survey of 157 Perth (Australia) hotel managers and their business colleagues confirmed the traditional view that the acute distress of gout can indeed be attributed to over-indulgence in alcohol, above all in beer.[17]

The more we drink, the less we appreciate our loss of skills thereby, as we lose the judgement and faculties which stamp us as individuals. Personality disorders attributable to alcoholism include a decline in intellectual ability, disturbance of memory and pathological changes in the brain. These effects place alcoholism among the most prominent causes of admissions to mental hospitals.[18]

A survey published in 1967 by the National Institute of Mental Health based on a study of 1343 alcoholics under treatment in San Francisco showed that accidents are seven times more likely to cause death among alcoholics than other people. Women with any of the personality traits, common among alcoholics, of invulnerability, feelings of omnipotence, depression and self-destructiveness were sixteen times more prone to accidents than other women.

A Public Health official in Chicago in 1967 also stated that deaths on the road due to drinking are not confined to drivers. A study of pedestrian deaths in Illinois that year showed that 42 per cent had been drinking. As for Mrs Barbara Castle's much maligned breath tests, it is known that road fatalities fell by 23 per cent in the last three months of 1967, and total casualties by 16 per cent following

---

* 1 oz provides about 170 calories, but is completely deficient in vitamins, minerals and proteins.

the implementation of the regulations. These facts speak for themselves, and should silence all selfishly biased critics of a restriction on personal habits, since they have already prevented the death and mutilation of many innocent people.   ,

Size of the problem in Britain

It was officially estimated in 1966 that between two to three million men and women in Britain drink to excess and therefore dangerously, with over half a million of these classifiable as alcoholics.[19] About a year later, *Medical Officer* published a report stating that alcoholism is a problem of important size though largely unrecognized in British industry, which is causing concern to doctors and sociologists, and the number of alcoholics admitted to mental hospitals had risen in the past few years. Thirty years ago, when the figures were far lower, a medical authority in the United States stated that 'if alcoholism were a communicable disease a national emergency would be declared'.[20] This dictum surely applies in the United Kingdom today, since the figure of over half a million only lists the actual sufferers and gives no clue to the vast numbers of other people involved. Like ink upset on blotting paper, a circle of darkness seeps outwards from the central victim, affecting family and friends in increasing misery and despair. What other illness bringing decay and death is so destructive of happiness in the home?

This is not a matter to be dealt with solely by the treatment centres provided by the State, necessary as these are. If alcoholics are to avail themselves of whatever treatment facilities are arranged, it is first absolutely essential to change the prevalent attitude among the general public. There should be no vestige of moral condemnation, lack of sympathy and even scorn, for someone who is a seriously ill person. Until this has been achieved, alcoholics will have added difficulty in admitting their condition, especially if still able to hold down a job and carry responsibility. We need a public health programme on the lines followed in the USA since 1944, disseminating facts sufficiently forcefully to dispel misconceptions, and to replace harmful with helpful attitudes among the general public. Indeed a beginning in this direction has now been made by the National Council on Alcoholism, but as a voluntary organization it seems to be short of adequate publicity, funds and support. It should be taken over by the Government to ensure that its aims are carried out as soon as possible. We all need to have our eyes forcibly opened to a very painful problem and we can all play a useful part, however small, in helping to find a solution.

De-glamorizing alcohol
In the United Kingdom education on the use of alcohol is said to be virtually non-existent. The National Council on Alcoholism is in favour of giving young people the facts on the subject, believing that in this way they will grow up to use this knowledge with judgement and discretion. Where restraints are rigidly imposed the tendency is to reach for forbidden fruit. They report a slow but increasing demand for information in the shape of enquiries from teenagers and undergraduates.

One of the most sensible pronouncements on the subject has come from the Assistant Professor of Psychiatry and Director of the Alcohol Clinic at Massachusetts General Hospital, Boston, USA, who told a New York Conference in 1967 that 'alcohol is here to stay, and people must learn to develop *a healthy attitude* to it'. It is difficult for instruction in the art of drinking to be given in the home owing to guilt feelings in many parents about their own drinking habits. However, his suggestion that these lessons should be given in schools, beginning say with wine diluted with water and gradually increasing in strength through school and on to university, seems rather less than practical. Soon after this suggestion the State Liquor Control Board in the USA, alarmed at the startling number of teenagers arrested for drunkenness, instituted a patrol to check the ages of customers in bars. This led the state of Pennsylvania, where there is state owner-ship of all off-licence shops, to begin an advertising campaign to persuade parents to sign a pledge that 'I am not going to let my children drink any alcoholic beverage at home or anywhere else before they are twenty-one'. A report issued some nine months later by the Co-operative Commission on the Study of Alcoholism seems to suggest that this was perhaps not the best way to go about it. The report suggested that the drinking age-limit should be brought down from twenty-one to eighteen, that there should be less social pressure to drink, and that advertisers should depict it in a family setting, since this was the 'relatively routine and unemotional manner' in which young people were introduced to alcohol in Chinese, Italian and Jewish families, where alcoholism is outstandingly rare.

Furthermore, the Alcoholic Division of the US Treasury refutes any claim that drink is good for you, that it has no harmful effects, that it leaves no hangover, that it will assist you to success, or improve the performance of athletes.

Clearly it is still necessary to devise some really acceptable way of achieving that 'healthy attitude to alcohol' which is at present conspicuously lacking in so many groups and spheres. We simply cannot afford to have half a million people suffer from the insidious and heart-breaking disease of alcoholism, and merely pass by on the other side.

Aiding the alcoholic

'The healthy body is a guest chamber for the mind, the sick a prison,' wrote Francis Bacon. Of all those imprisoned in a sick body there can be few more in need of our aid and sympathy than the alcoholic, who can be helped and is as worthy of help as any other victim of disease. How can this aid best be given? This is primarily a public health problem, because it is an illness involving not only families but employers, fellow employees, social workers, clergy and even strangers. We must all support and make widely known the views of Dr Lincoln Williams, President of the National Council on Alcoholism, that 'there is need for greater research, more specialized treatment, better aftercare facilities, and the imperative need to bring home to the public that alcoholism is a *treatable disease*'. He does not fail to emphasize that there is still *no cure, that the only chance of recovery for an alcoholic is to forswear alcohol forever*.[21] Meanwhile a gift of £100,000 in 1968 for research to the Medical Council on Alcoholism from an anonymous body will no doubt assist in throwing light on some aspects of the problem.

Treatment

Being highly specialized, treatment is something only doctors can give. It is practically always necessary, for spontaneous cures are rare, and are generally a sequel of religious conversion, not usual in this day and age. Alcoholics often persist in claiming, while failing repeatedly to do so, that they can give it up of their own accord if they want to. Unfortunately, there is a great shortage of doctors equipped by knowledge or sympathy to cope with such patients as can summon up enough courage to risk a rebuff or lack of understanding if they approach them for advice and aid. Greater attention to the whole subject will no doubt be given in the medical training schools of the future or even today. They might well extend their activities to include refresher courses for older men wishing to enlarge their, at present, very limited knowledge in this pressing field.

It now seems probable that work carried out by Dr Pierre Marie de Go on 50,000 male alcoholics in one million examinations and reported by him to a Medical Conference on Alcoholism in 1967 could ultimately reach a point where a computer could handle his tables for detecting incipient alcoholism. It seems possible that this might lead to such an early diagnosis that there might be some large-scale prevention of a disease now afflicting 13 per cent of French males aged from twenty to fifty-five years, and a smaller but increasing number of British citizens. Help must also be offered by everyone of us for, directly or indirectly, alcoholism concerns us all. But the patient has to make the first move. No one can do anything for him until he can admit that he is floundering, and is in dire need.

For many this is such an unbearable admission that it cannot be made until the uttermost depths have been plumbed. Being no longer master of himself but a slave, he may and often does loathe his slavery, and lament inwardly with Cassio that man should put an enemy in his mouth to steal away his brains. He has got to a state where he cannot face life without his fetters. He either pretends they do not exist, or goes 'on the wagon' to demonstrate his freedom. Unfortunately, he always returns to his slavery. However, no one enjoys slavery, least of all the sensitive and highly intelligent, so often among the enslaved, plunged in unfathomable gulfs of guilt and self-disgust that none but a fellow victim can conceive.

Nor is the alcoholic the only one to take refuge in unreality. There is a mistaken loyalty in the family or groups to which he belongs that says, 'Let's not look, and this will disappear.' Concealment helps no one. Every single case deserves concern and compassion, but must first be openly acknowledged. The uninformed and outdated method of ignoring any case of TB in the hope that it will go away has disappeared. The same commonsense attitude should apply to alcoholism.

For the alcoholic himself, 'the first essential step, without which no progress is possible, is for the alcoholic to realize that he is an alcoholic,' wrote Raymond Blackburn, once an eminent Member of Parliament, in his book *I am an Alcoholic* published in 1960. Giving a factual account of the despair, degradation and ruin that overwhelmed him in mid-career owing to the addiction that brands the disease, he detailed the onset, progress in deterioration and eventual containment of his illness. He earns our respect for having laid bare his sufferings and darkened soul in the hope that his history might help others to salvation.

Salvation through total future abstinence. This is the one hope and promise held out by Alcoholics Anonymous (AA), whose instant response to any cry for help has saved so many from despair. This amazing organization of men and women was founded in Ohio in 1935 by a doctor and a stockbroker, and is still run entirely by and for recovered and recovering alcoholics. It now numbers well over 250,000 in about 1000 groups in more than fifty countries, with 450 groups now in Britain.* Unfortunately, this represents only a tiny minority of those needing the help it offers to all willing to accept the very simple conditions laid down. Every member is committed to learning how to find and then how to maintain sobriety through total abstinence for the rest of life, and so become self-rehabilitated and able to resume an ordinary and useful existence. The only requirement for membership is the desire to stop drinking. Largely because it is based on the principle that the best way to help one's self is to help others, it remains a rock on which thousands have rebuilt their shattered lives.

Alcoholism being a family disease,[22] though there is no evidence of genetic inheritance of alcoholism,[23] the personal and social misery it causes cannot be adequately assessed. These remain vastly greater than any figures of admissions to hospitals or treatment centres can possibly indicate. Years of life with an alcoholic make whole families ill from fear, shame, irritability and anxiety, as well as from the insecurity that dogs the deterioration of the bread-winner. Things go from bad to worse, until—in the fortunate cases—he gets adequate medical treatment and aftercare, and/or joins AA. Now, at last, he is committed to remaining 'dry' for ever. But this does not mean the end of his troubles. The struggle to maintain sobriety may be terrible. Resentment, self-pity and jittery nerves have become habitual, and debts have grown tangible and pressing. So wives and families also stand in aid of learning new physical, mental and spiritual habits, if they too are to reach new levels of health and harmony.

This assistance has also been provided by AA who issue a helpful booklet of do's and don'ts for their special enlightenment, and

* According to a report by AA issued on 23 September 1971 there has been an increase of over 300 groups in the last ten years, reflecting not so much a growth of alcoholism but a recognition of an illness.

encourage the formation of Al-Anon groups for the wives and relatives of alcoholics held simultaneously with the regular and frequent 'dry' gatherings of local AA groups which are so valuable in keeping members sober together, and able to enjoy some social life unplagued by temptations to drink again.

Even if their particular alcoholic has not joined AA, free consultations are now given for the families in this country by the National Council on Alcoholism established in 1962. This has its own programme for fighting the disease and has help available for families, friends and employers.

Cheap nutritional aids for alcoholics and their families
Alcoholism devours money as well as happiness in the home. Standards of living have usually been reduced to a very low level before the compulsive drinking stops and with it the outlay of money on alcohol. But there are two very important food factors which should be budgeted for in every case, if at all possible. These are vitamin B complex and vitamin C because all these people need this extra help, and it should be given priority.

Since alcohol consists entirely of calories from carbohydrates with no content of minerals or vitamins, all 'dry' alcoholics start on their difficult way of abstinence with a huge backlog of deficiency of vitamin B complex, and especially of thiamine (vitamin B_1) and riboflavin (vitamin B_2). These are needed to metabolize (break down) the pyruvic acid from incompletely broken-down carbohydrates which is flooding the tissues, so as to make it available as a source of energy for the body and mind. It has even been found that cases of alcoholic coma can be restored to consciousness by a large injection of vitamin B_1. This is emergency medical treatment only, and multiple deficiencies of other members of the complex have been caused by long periods on vitamin B_1 alone, for their action is synergistic (working together). The deficiency is best overcome by taking a good food source of the whole B complex such as brewer's yeast.

All alcoholics, including those who have gone 'dry' as well as those of their wives who have not given up the sugars and 'secret sugars' denounced in the next chapter, would benefit by taking daily from one teaspoon to one tablespoon of powdered brewer's yeast in a little water with each meal. It is a by-product of brewing, containing no alcohol, and is an excellent source of vitamin B complex. It is also an effective laxative, so if the stools later become over-loose the amount taken should be reduced.

From personal experience as a voluntary worker with members of Al-Anon in a group of AA in a Cape Town suburb, I have found that husbands who at first refused to take the yeast, became willing to do so after seeing the good effects on the energy, appearance, moods and temper of their wives, for it works to quieten the nervous system, improve the vitality and restore the optimum weight. A letter received from one such wife contains the following lines. 'I have been feeding D. now on your brewer's yeast for six months and he is a different person. For the first time in his life he is putting on weight, and gets up in the morning and says, "I've never felt so fit in my life." '

The heavy stress on both alcoholics and their families needs to be compensated by extra large amounts of vitamin C. Where a garden is available this can be obtained by daily salads freshly prepared from any freshly shredded greenleaf vegetables especially cabbage, red and white, broccoli flowers, grated turnips and beets (all far better sources than lettuces) tossed in oil and sprinkled with lemon juice to preserve the vitamin C content. Flat dwellers can grow mustard and cress on window sills and sprout wheat as cheap sources of this valuable vitamin.

Attitude of employers

Because managements do not understand that 'alcoholism is a disease, and there is a disease called alcoholism' they remain unconvinced that they undergo considerable financial losses through the prevalence of problem drinkers among their staffs, although the firm's directors may be aware of them. While precise figures are not available, a study by WHO in the UN reported between 300,000 and 500,000 alcoholics costing the country some £40 million every year in the form of days lost, loss of operating efficiency and production, as well as in misplaced judgements and resignations on the plea of ill-health.[24]

One of the avowed aims of the AA is to encourage special alcohol programmes throughout industry so as to 'eliminate this immense wastage of time, material, money, goodwill and health and human life itself', and it publishes a number of informative leaflets and will supply further information on application.

Another organization, National Lifeline, a consortium consisting of the Helping Hand Organization, the Apex Trust and the Circle

Trust has published its own report expressing similar aims on 'Alcoholism in Industry'. This is available on application. It points out that in the USA, where alcoholism is estimated to cost the country two billion dollars yearly, there are 250 companies employing altogether some six million people which have each laid down a company policy on alcoholism. This entails treating it as a disease and allowing sick leave for treatment. The recovery rate as a result of this enlightened approach has reached from 60 to 75 per cent and one company has saved some 750,000 dollars a year in sick leave alone.[25]

Any employer could well take a lesson from the British Civil Service on how best to avoid this loss among some of their most valued employees who are heading for disaster from compulsive drinking. Provisions made for treating them at a National Health Service Centre include normal sick leave, with an added rehabilitation period if necessary, and the department also permits part-time attendance or makes a transfer to some other department if this is in the best interests of the patient. If treatment is not successful, staff may be retired on the grounds of ill-health, as for any other illness, with no sacrifice of pension rights.[26]

The great importance of a personal reaction on our part of understanding and acceptance rather than that of censure, frivolous mockery or disbelief, is shown by the wonderful success of AA. The statement, 'Sorry, I can't take a drink', should evoke no more comment and certainly no more hostility than such another statement as, 'Sorry, I'm allergic to apples.' Drinks should be offered but a refusal accepted as normal. Anyone struggling to climb the slippery slopes of the twelve steps of AA, or groping along the harder way of going it alone, should be made to feel free to speak of his illness naturally, instead of trying to cover it up. His friends and others must learn not to conceal liquor from him; not to surreptitiously spike a chosen soft drink, and not to press him to have just one—to toast the bride, or whatever. Especially among social drinkers there seems to be some misunderstanding about these recommendations. It must be repeated as forcefully as possible that while there is no known cure, one basic fact about alcoholism is known without a shadow of doubt. This is that the only way for an alcoholic to arrest his disease – and only he can do this—is to stop drinking alcohol, and never to drink it again. It is as simple, yet as supremely difficult for him, as that. He needs all the help we can give him. Above all, we should never, never try to persuade an alcoholic that he is not an alcoholic, for this may mean death to him. It is an act of barbarous cruelty to offer him even *one* drink. He must *never* drink again.

Alcoholism must be considered a pressing problem for the Public Health authorities, the medical profession and the community, and we do not yet know how it can be prevented. What we do know is that we must all of us open our eyes and hearts to a problem which may seem far from us individually, but should always remain a matter of concern for us all, since as John Donne has said, 'No man is an island, entire of itself . . . every man's death diminisheth me, for I am involved in mankind.'

REFERENCES

1 JELLINEK, E. M., MD. *The Disease Concept of Alcoholism* (Hillhouse Press, Newhaven, Conn., 1961)
2 KESSEL, NEIL, MD, WALTON, HENRY, MD. *Alcoholism* (Penguin Books, 1965)
3 MOSS, M. C., MB, BS, DPM, DAVIES, E. BERESFORD, MD, DPM. *A Survey of Alcoholism in an English County* (By courtesy of Geigy (UK) Limited Pharmaceuticals Division, 1967)
4 RAYMOND, E. V. *et al.* 'Chronic Alcoholism in Paris', *Arch. Mal. Prof.*, 21, 413–27 (1960)
5 KESSEL, NEIL, MD, WALTON, HENRY, MD. *Alcoholism* (Penguin Books, 1965)
6 *Ibid.*
7 MALZBERG, B. *The Alcoholic Psychosis* (The Free Press, 1960)
8 WILLIAMS, ROGER *et al.* Proc. *US. Nat. Acad. Science*, 56, 566 (1966)
9 MAENPAA, P. H. *et al.* *Quart. Jour. Studies on Alcohol.*, 27, 596–603 (1966)
10 FORBES, J. C. *et al.* *Quart. Jour. Studies on Alcohol*
11 KESSEL, NEIL, MD, and WALTON, HENRY, MD. *Alcoholism* (Penguin Books, 1965)
12 *Ibid.*
13 *Ibid.*
14 *Ibid.*
15 *Ibid.*
16 *Ibid.*
17 REILLY, K. A. *et al. Medical Jour. of Australia*, No. 1, 1213 (1967)
18 LEMERE, F. *Am. J. Psych.*, 113, 361 (1956)
19 KEMP, ROBERT, MD. *Drinking and Alcoholism* (BMA, 1966)
20 MENNINGER, WILLIAM, MD. *Man Against Himself* (Harcourt Brace, New York, 1938)
21 WILLIAMS, LINCOLN, MD, *et al. The Practitioner* (1 February 1968)
22 JACKSON, JOAN, K. PHD, *Quart. Jour. Studies on Alcohol*, 15, 562–85 (1954)
23 KESSEL, NEIL, MD, and WALTON, HENRY, MD. *Alcoholism* (Penguin Books, 1965)
24 *Alcoholism in Industry* (Published by National Lifeline, 25 Camberwell Grove, London, SE5)

25   NATIONAL COUNCIL ON ALCOHOLISM, 212a Shaftesbury Avenue, London, WC2
26   *Alcoholism in Industry* (Published by National Life Line, 28 Camberwell Grove, London, SE5)

USEFUL ADDRESSES

GREAT BRITAIN

a   ALCOHOLICS ANONYMOUS, 11 Redcliffe Gardens, London, SW10. Phone: Flaxman 9669 (Addresses of local groups and all AA publications on request)
b   NATIONAL COUNCIL ON ALCOHOLISM, 212a Shaftesbury Avenue, London, WC2 (Free consultations and many inexpensive publications)
c   NATIONAL LIFELINE, 25 Camberwell Grove, London, SE5 (Leaflet *Alcoholism in Industry* free on application)
d   THE LONDON ALCOHOLISM INFORMATION CENTRE, 25a Wincott Street, London, SE11
e   GLASGOW COUNCIL ON ALCOHOLISM, 141 Bath Street, Glasgow

AUSTRALIA
NEW SOUTH WALES

a   ALCOHOLICS ANONYMOUS, 81 York Street, Sydney 2000
b   ALCOHOLISM RESEARCH FOUNDATION, 194 Pitt Street, Sydney 2000
c   ALCOHOLISM INFORMATION CENTRE, Langton Clinic, Dowling Street, Moore Park, Sydney 2000
d   DIVISION OF ESTABLISHMENTS, The Director, Department of Public Service, 9–13 Young Street, Sydney 2000

QUEENSLAND

a   ALCOHOLICS ANONYMOUS, 80A Wickham Fortitude Valley, Brisbane
b   THE DEPARTMENT OF HEALTH, Administration Building, George and Elizabeth Streets, Brisbane

SOUTH AUSTRALIA

a   ALCOHOLICS ANONYMOUS, 101 Angus Street, Adelaide 5000
b   ALCOHOL AND DRUG ADDICTS (TREATMENT) BOARD, 198 North Terrace, Adelaide 5000

TASMANIA

a   ALCOHOLICS ANONYMOUS, Bathurst Street, Hobart
b   ALCOHOLISM INFORMATION CENTRE, 429 Elizabeth Street, Hobart

VICTORIA

a   ALCOHOLICS ANONYMOUS, Town Hall Chambers, 246 Little Collins Street, Melbourne 3000
b   ALCOHOLISM FOUNDATION OF VICTORIA, 105 Collins Street, Melbourne 3000

WEST AUSTRALIA

a   ALCOHOLICS ANONYMOUS, 76 Murray Street, Perth 6000
b   REHABILITATION CENTRE, The Commissioner, Public Health Dept., Murray Street, Perth 6000

U.S.A.

a   NATIONAL COUNCIL ON ALCOHOLISM INC., New York Academy of Medicine Building, 2 East 103rd Street, New York 29, New York

b   GENERAL SERVICE BOARD OF ALCOHOLICS ANONYMOUS INC., PO Box 439, Grand Central Annex, New York 17, New York (Addresses of local groups supplied on application)

CANADA

a   CANADIAN FEDERATION ON ALCOHOLIC PROBLEMS, 11 Prince Arthur Avenue, Toronto 5, Ontario

b   ALCOHOLICS ANONYMOUS, 733 Raches East, Montreal, Quebec

NEW ZEALAND

a   NATIONAL SOCIETY ON ALCOHOLISM INC., Paragon Chambers, Welburn Avenue, Wellington 1

b   ALCOHOLISM TRUST BOARD, 140 Symonds Street, Auckland 1

c   ALCOHOLICS ANONYMOUS, 78 Albert Street, Auckland 1

SOUTH AFRICA

a   NATIONAL COUNCIL ON ALCOHOLISM, 319/320 Charter House, 13 Rissik Street, PO Bag 10134, Johannesburg

b   ALCOHOLICS ANONYMOUS, Service Information Centre, PO Box 1324, Pretoria (Addresses of local groups supplied on application. Addresses of treatment centres provided by the State obtainable from any local hospital, magistrate or Social Welfare Office)

9

The Sweet Life

'Much of our present dietary trouble arises from the fact that 200 years ago man learnt how to isolate sugar.'

PROFESSOR JOHN YUDKIN

The compulsive drinking of alcoholism ranks among the most dangerous addictions of man; less serious in its effects, but adversely affecting many more millions, is the modern addiction to sugar.

The most valuable gift a fairy godmother could bring to a modern christening would be an anti-sweet tooth. In nature sweetness is a *flavour* not an emasculated *food*, robbing the natural appetite so that we eat less of the essential proteins and vegetables since these no longer seem sufficiently attractive to a palate addicted to sweetness. In fact, possessing a sweet tooth has become one of the direst curses of civilized races. So, as fairies do not get invitations to functions today, it is clearly up to us humans to try instead to stem the flood of sugar which threatens to swamp us with obesity, diabetes, latent heart disease, dental decay, asthma, catarrh, low blood sugar, and a host of lesser ills.

The Cocoa, Chocolate and Confectionery Alliance estimated that in 1965 the cost of our consumption of chocolate and sugar confectionery was nearly £298 million, averaging 7·5 oz. a week per person.[1] This shows that Britain spent more on sweets that year than any other nation for which figures are available. We have, it seems, even overtaken the white South Africans with their average annual sugar consumption of 121 lbs per person, and the Americans with theirs of 100 lbs. Far behind these lag the French with a figure of only 66 lbs; and they enjoy a high life expectancy rate of seventy years. What could give a clearer pointer to the unpleasant fact that as a nation we have reached a degree of addiction that can only be described as sheer twentieth-century slavery? How much further must we slide downhill from the moderation—the one great blessing of war-time rationing—which compelled us all to eat less sugar?

We do not know when sugar began to exercise its sinister power over man, for its use in Asia antedates authentic history, though the name is said to have its origin in the Sanscrit word 'Sakkara'. It remained, however, a rare and precious commodity brought in the eighth century by Arab traders to Sicily and Spain, and taken later by Columbus to the West Indies. In the reign of Queen Elizabeth I it was still regarded as a costly condiment, priced at the equivalent of £2 for a pound. Today when it is, unfortunately, so comparatively cheap and so plentiful, it has earned the stern condemnation of responsible physicians, dentists and nutritionists everywhere. As Dr Philip M. Lowell wrote recently in the *Los Angeles Times*, 'Sugar is the most injurious product in the national dietary, with no exception, and under every possible condition—it is the ultimate in food degeneration because all life has been removed.'

The last sentence holds the full irony of the situation. The untreated stem of the sugar cane is a nutritious source of carbohydrate, containing all the vitamins and minerals necessary to convert it into energy in the body of the eater who can cope with this, if sufficient energy is expended. During treatment, short lengths of this cane are crushed to express a blackish juice known as molasses and mostly sold as cattle feed, while the crystallized portion of crude sugar is sold as Muscovado or Barbados after evaporation in open pans. The main part of the product is further refined to produce white sugar, and it is in this processing that all the vitamins and minerals are removed, so that what is commonly consumed is even more devoid of life than the Dead Sea. As Sir Robert McCarrison emphasized years ago, 'Man cannot build up living tissue from materials which have in themselves no necessary connection with living protoplasm.'

The great white lie

Few carefully built-up images can be so false as that of white sugar, promoted as so pleasant, so stable, so concentrated and so 'pure'. All quite true, no doubt, especially when 'pureness' is recognized as meaning 'absence of life'. There is no mention of the really salient facts that it contains no vitamins, a mere smear of minerals, and will support no form of life. Its real nature has earned for it the title of 'The Great White Lie' in the opinion of Dr Carlton Fredericks.[2]

What reaches us as white sugar, beginning as a perfectly good natural food in highly concentrated form, has not only been deprived of its food value, but has been turned into a thief itself, stealing vitamin B_1 in the body from other more reputable foods in order to become available as a source of energy.

In her book *Red Strangers*, Elspeth Huxley, Kenya born and bred, refers to the habit of the Kikuyu mother working in the field, of giving some sugar cane to her child to suck, as food and drink in one. Indeed, in this, its original form, before it has been robbed by refinement, it is highly nutritious, and is so used by workers in cane brakes the world over. Even when it has been reduced to black strap molasses it remains a good source of calcium (258 mg per 100 grams), iron (7·97 mg per 100 grams) and copper (1·93 mg per 100 grams).[3] But when it has undergone the full treatment it has become an insidious enemy, and this is growing more and more evident to the medical and dental world.

Roughly the same procedure is followed with sugar beet—the nutritious portion going as cattle feed, and the waste product being sold for human consumption. In their masterly *Diabetes, Coronary Thrombosis and the Saccharine Diseases*[4] Drs Cleave and Campbell have pinpointed the fact that Indian cane-cutters around Durban chew enormous quantities of cane as they carry out the most strenuous jobs in the world handicapped by a moist hot climate and yet suffer no ill effects. Other Indians working nearby in far lighter capacities but eating a far smaller amount of refined white sugar become diabetics in large numbers.

Nor are ill effects confined to what is obviously seen to be sugar. They result also from the 'secret sugars' commonly consumed in sweets, chocolates, biscuits, cakes, breakfast cereals, ices, bottled drinks, pastries, pies, etc. According to the Ministry of Labour *Gazette* for 1966, the average household spent 34p. a week on biscuits and cake, but only 32½p. on vegetables, excluding potatoes, which accounted for another 18p. Only 30p. was spent on bread, being rather less than on cake and biscuits, which seems to throw an odd light on the much-quoted remark of Marie Antoinette. In fact, we in Britain might be said to suffer from a perpetual blight of biscuits, since we lead the world in the number we consume each year.

It is absolute rubbish to claim, as so many do, that 'we must have sugar to give us energy' (*pace* Dr Eric Trimmer in the Family Doctor's booklet *Getting Married*) when the term 'sugar' is taken to mean the waste product remaining when the valuable juices of the sugar cane have been so treated that they have been stripped of all their minerals and vitamins, leaving nothing but concentrated calories. This product should be termed 'sucrose', and according to Professor Yudkin of London University, 'The body simply does not need sucrose.'[5] A hundred grams of sucrose require 0·18 milligrams of vitamin B_1 to convert itself into the glucose which is the only form in which it can be absorbed in the body. Since all the vitamin B_1 previously present was removed during the processing, it is forced to steal this vitamin from other foods eaten. If no surplus is available it proceeds to flood the tissues with unconverted pyruvic acid which steals vitamin B and blocks the assimilation of calcium, causing at first such common complaints as shortness of breath, pains in joints and muscles, stiffness from coalescing of proteins, and general unfitness, and later more serious disabilities.

Never touching white sugar, or any of the 'secret sugars', we can all get all the energy-giving glucose we need in the most active of lives, for nearly 70 per cent of unprocessed food of any origin that we eat or drink can be converted in the body into glucose and then stored as glycogen, mostly in the liver, for future use as required. The added sense of well-being has to be experienced to be credited.

Sugar spells Slaughter

It could justly be claimed that 'Sugar spells Slaughter'. Taken in excess, as it is in so many homes and in all innocence, it is the chief enemy of a slim supple alert body, good teeth, a lively mind, a healthy skin, sweet temper and a long and healthy life. This is no new knowledge, for an old Scottish saw warns us that

> '*With sugar bestrewn*
> *Old age is no boon.*'

Or may never be reached at all, according to some expert opinion.

Professor John Yudkin of Queen Elizabeth College, London, has been awarded a grant of £9000 by the Heart Foundation to carry out diet trials to test his theory that one cause of coronary thrombosis may be excessive sugar in the diet. He has pointed out that this is an affliction of affluence, associated with a greater intake of sugar occurring with greater wealth, and suggests that the hypothesis that this is a major cause of a disease killing 100,000 yearly in Britain alone deserves to be tested by intensive research equal to the tremendous amount devoted to the high fat hypothesis, which has not been conclusively established.

Today even our pets consume excess sugar and pay the price. Some years ago the city of Toronto, famous for its Dr Banting who won the Nobel Prize for his insulin discoveries, started a clinic to help dogs suffering from diabetes and many now have daily injections of insulin. Symptoms of diabetes in one dog, however, cleared up as soon as the owner took the clinic's advice and stopped feeding it a pound of toffee every week! Publicity was also given to the sad case of Sir Winston Churchill's famous poodle Rufus, who eventually landed at the surgery of a well-known veterinarian. Here he was described as being 'very plump and lethargic, and his teeth in an awful state'. It seems that his master, who loved chocolates, always shared them with Rufus. The spoilt dog, who had lost most of his teeth, was put on a sensible diet, and one hopes he duly recovered his slimness and energy.

As for children's teeth today, the threatened fluoridation of water is an attempt by the authorities to deal with a condition that in the opinion of many experts would be far more wisely dealt with by cutting consumption of sweets and 'secret sugars'. In fact, the President of the British Dental Association once went so far as to announce that 'if all sweet shops were prohibited by law, the dentist's work with children would largely disappear'. There seems no chance of this reform, though a few enlightened schools have ordained that apples should replace biscuits for the mid-morning break, but there are still thousands of others where nothing is being done. This is surely a matter where it is up to each parent and each Parent Teacher Association to act firmly. Dental treatment is free but that is no reason for accepting the necessity for dentures at an early age.

Insurance against a short life
The best insurance against a short life and a sugary one is to make a good choice of parents. The ways in which we are brought up have an extraordinary hold on us, and there are vast numbers of adults who hate any thought of change, like silkworms that starve rather than eat anything but mulberry leaves. So that training for change—to be able to regard nothing but love as immutable, and any alteration as an adventure—cannot be established too early in life. Nutritionists are agreed that a considerable variety of food can and should be introduced to children as young as under one year. Providing the food is suitable, they like this and can cope with it. The best technique is to combine a new food with one already popular, and to vary it in

form with as many or more savoury as sweet flavours. To say plaintively, 'My child won't eat peas, porridge, raw fruit, or what-have-you', is an admission of defeat and lack of imagination that should not be made. Hunger is still the best sauce, and a healthy happy child should be a hungry child, never pushed to eat more than he needs or wants.

Gone, fortunately, are the days of Glaxo babies with their rolls of fat at wrist and ankle, but, alas, 'biscuit babies' and 'sugar children' are still with us. During the seven years in which I ran a physio-therapy clinic for an LCC Welfare Centre dealing with under-fives, I had plenty of opportunity for detecting these, and there were many. The fact that I would accuse the mother of feeding sweets and/or biscuits in large amounts to the child in question soon gained me the reputation of a witch. The only witchcraft I had used was a gentle, unobserved pinch which revealed the flabby flesh resulting from those unhealthy habits, but it proved a useful reputation, and a great help in getting strict injunctions to 'ban the biscuits, and stop the sweets' carried out. In view of the large number of cases of enlarged tonsils so common today it is interesting to recall that as long ago as 1923 it was found that high sugar content in food caused the tonsils of kittens to enlarge to twice the normal size.

Possible sources of the craving
If the body does not indeed need sucrose, why this evident craving? Firstly, it seems to be due to habit, established all too often in infancy with baby foods replacing breast feeding,[6] then to injudicious choice of first foods, and such supplements as sweetened orange juice. Now, one small orange contains nearly as much starch as three small new potatoes, and certainly tastes sweet enough for any unperverted palate. Yet it has been sweetened. Surely some better method of preservation could be found?

Next comes early childhood when doting grandparents and other equally misguided adults bring offerings of sweets, chocolates, biscuits, lollies, ices and so on. Why in the name of Nicholas, patron saint of children, has no one taught us that these should only be eaten (if at all) in strictest moderation and only with meals, never between whiles? Why do we not offer, and share, raisins, dates (in moderation), nuts, apples, well-scrubbed young carrots, beets and turnips, etc., crisp strips of leaves of green or red cabbage, sticks of celery and bite-sized bits of cheese? I have many, many times proved that all these will be enthusiatically received. With good chewing by young jaws eager for exercise, they not only give equal pleasure and a taste of sweetness as the saliva breaks down the starch, but start the new generation on the way it should travel, with no sense of deprivation, and keep the teeth that no artificial substitutes can ever adequately replace.

Then comes school, with the road to the tuck shop or confectioner practically paved with the decayed or lost teeth of their youthful customers. At this stage we need active Parent Teacher Associations to take a hand in the necessary reforms. Of course this must be a matter of keeping in line with the practice in the home or it will have little value.

In teenagers undergoing the physical and psychological strains of adolescence the effects of the sweet life of sugar addiction generally shows itself in a pasty complexion studded with acne spots. Since this affliction may add pounds to the heavy burden of self-consciousness already carried at this age, it can be a real cause of unacknowledged distress. Somehow, we need to get them to give up the ointments and lotions they buy in vain, and get them on to a balanced diet, with no sugars—white or 'secret'. In three months this should have proved its worth, but it must naturally be continued or the trouble will return throughout young adulthood. Since there is usually a high degree of offending material still requiring conversion into energy, it is useful to add one to four teaspoons of debittered brewers' yeast stirred into a little water and taken with meals until the complexion has cleared.

Perhaps the sugar habit even has you by the heart—and this may be literally true, for the heart muscles like any others are irritated and waterlogged by unbroken down pyruvic acid, retarding the pulse far below normal. How can you hope to break away? Frankly, only by resolve and perseverance. It is so much easier to turn to some 'miracle drug' than to try to throw out habits that seem to be built into the very structure of daily life. But it is this 'vital habit of breaking habits' as J. B. S. Haldane called it, which we have to acquire somehow. Slavery to sugar, or any other addiction for that matter, is no case for legislation. We need no Wilberforce to shock us, only our own will-power to stiffen us. It is not easy to break these habits, probably sustained for many years. 'We have need,' to quote the late Dr Weston Price, 'for a strength of character and will-power such as will make us use the things our bodies require, rather than the foods we like.'[7] It is comforting to reflect that, given time, we not only do not miss the things we have given up, but prefer the new ones. The war taught us that we all possess reserves of resolution of mind and action however deeply these may lie hidden. Here is another war against hurtful habits in which we can call upon these reserves to fight the battle against waste. For surely it is gross waste to fritter away the stores of energy, health and joyfulness we might have for the taking.

Should you, or those for whom you provide food, complain that without sugar the world seems robbed for its sweets, I would reply with Petulengro, 'There's night and day, brother, both sweet things,' likewise all the natural sugars in fruit, vegetables, meats, fish, eggs, milk and its products; and each of these (if unprocessed) contains the vitamins necessary for its complete conversion into food, not flotsam, for the body.

Once the resolve has been taken, whether by one's self alone, or by all of the family at once, the sensible way seems to be to start by substituting for sugar such good sources of sweetness as honey, molasses, raisins, figs, etc., as well, of course, as plenty of fruit and fruit juices. A word of caution here. In a new-found enthusiasm for honey, it is advisable not to go as far as this anonymous writer:

> *I eat my peas with honey,*
> *I've done it all my life.*
> *It makes the peas taste funny,*
> *But it keeps them on the knife.*

Nor should we merely replace the banned substance while repeating the bulk and frequency. I encountered this method in a firmly teetotal member of Alcoholics Anonymous who drank frequent glasses of milk well-laced with molasses, instead of glasses of brandy, then wondered why her weight continued to go up rather than down. Honey, like all forms of concentrated food, is high in calories and must be used in strict moderation. Incidentally, ripe fruit of any kind, cooked only briefly and briskly with the lid on, becomes quite acceptable to even the sweet-toothed if served with the top of the milk into which a tablespoon of non-instant skim milk has been whisked, giving the slightly sweetish flavour of milk sugar.

As for back-sliding occasionally, if you feel you must eat just one sweet or chocolate between meals, i.e. on an empty stomach, drink a glass of water at the same time to dilute it. Undiluted sugar is hydroscopic, puckering the cheek when held against it in sucking, and irritating the mucus membrane, which may lead to catarrh.

Finally, we should all remember that Food Reform, however worthy, is only a means to a better life, not an end in itself, and should always remain an objective, not an obsession.

Blood sugar levels
While in diabetes there is too much sugar in the blood, the opposite condition can cause such common ailments as fatigue, restlessness, tension, headaches, irritability, depression (the 'vile melancholy' of Dr Johnson) and inability to concentrate. Paradoxically enough, this low blood sugar arises from eating too much sugar, which is devoured avidly when the level is low, but is not wanted if the level is normal. Sugar boosts the blood sugar initially and gives a transient feeling of relief, but by stimulating the pancreas to pour out insulin too quickly and too much, the blood sugar is burnt up rapidly.

The liver is also over-stimulated and therefore does its job too zealously, putting too much away into storage as glycogen, and the end result is again a low blood sugar level. More sugar is then taken and the vicious circle is repeated. The lower the blood level falls, the lower the morale. Since it is known that the nicotine in smoking, and the caffeine in strong tea, black coffee, and some widely sold bottled drinks have the same apparently lifting, but ultimately lowering, result through their effect on the adrenals, they fall under the same taboo.

Deliberately giving up sugar can be as difficult as giving up cigarettes and to do both seems to demand well nigh impossible standards of determination. Yet it has been done many, many times with nothing but the happiest of results. It seems that if half the energy that is put into acquiring harmful habits is put into defeating them, we really get somewhere. Of course the motivation must be strong enough. Film and TV stars have insisted on having health food shops in Los Angeles—obviously their occupation puts a very high premium on unfailing good health and good looks.

Glucose or blood sugar is as important to life as oxygen itself, but as we breathe in oxygen we burn up our blood sugar which must be kept up to a certain pitch minute by minute to allow the brain to function properly. This explains the feeling of mental inability and brain fatigue commonly found among sugar addicts. Again, such minor ills as shortness of breath and excess sweating on exertion can be traced to excess sugar. Oxygen being required for its combustion, sugar uses up the oxygen needed for muscle work, so that exercising generates too much heat. The breathing becomes shallow if, in the absence of sufficient vitamin B_1, the sugar eaten is not oxidized beyond the stage of pyruvic acid, since not enough carbon dioxide is given out to stimulate the breathing centre correctly. Deep breathing and ease in exercise, therefore, depend on less sugar being taken into the body. So here is another benefit to be obtained by cutting it out, or down very drastically to begin with.

We can but echo the wish of an eminent American physician that 'instead of the popular explosion into the field of heart diseases, some of our bright young men should take up as a life work the study of nutrition', since this would lay the emphasis on methods of prevention rather than on patching up damage often committed in sheer ignorance. For the present it seems to be the responsibility of the housewife to heed the advice and knowledge of the small numbers of great figures of their followers in this field. That wise philosopher Whitehead believed that 'the worth of a man lies in his liability to persuasion'. Perhaps we can all be persuaded to try out a period with *no sugar* and *all whole foods*. If after four to eight weeks we feel no different (and this is highly unlikely), we shall at least have given it a go, and can return unconverted to our old ways.

Artificial sweeteners

Giving up the sweet life of slavery to sugar, however, could do no one any possible harm, and might indeed do him or her a power of good. On no account, however, should anyone turn to sugar substitutes which may be more undesirable still. For instance, commercial glucose is manufactured by the action on corn starch of sulphur dioxide which was known to be harmful as long ago as the fifteenth century, and is regarded today as definitely deleterious by authorities in the USA, but it is still much in use in soft drinks.

Nor should we forget that our own great nutritionist, the late Sir Jack Drummond, warned us against a couple of synthetic sweeteners commonly employed in this way and in food, yet they continued in favour for many years following his warning. Saccharine, popularly supposed to be quite permissible since it is recommended to diabetics, is a coal tar derivative and therefore suspect as a carcinogen of long-term effect, and it is a protoplasmic poison forbidden in some countries, but still allowed in Britain. In fact, it was the only synthetic sweetener legally permitted up to 1960, as rats could eat it with impunity.

Slimmers, especially, should be on their guard against any new and artfully advertised substance that could do them no good. It seems that food manufacturers have discovered that as more overweighters get calorie-conscious there will be an expanding market for low calorie substitutes for sugar. It should prove a highly profitable affair, for them, if not for the consumer. Whatever the reason, high pressure salesmanship of sugarless sweeteners has hit these shores with a bang. The slogans and sweeteners are bursting out of the chemists' shops into wider windows, but there seems little reason to suppose that what was once regarded as a wolf can now be looked at as a lamb, whatever its clothing.

The controversy over cyclamates, permitted for the artificial sweetening of soft drinks and confectionery, received a great deal of attention in the Press. It seems worthwhile pointing out that in the USA the National Research Council warned against their use in 1955 and again in 1962, saying that their safety could not be guaranteed.[8] Anyone taking such drinks may consume as much as a teaspoon of cyclamate daily[9] which is known to destroy vitamin C,[10] and there are physicians who believe that cyclamates may cause serious liver damage.[11]

The British Industrial Biological Research Association has been carrying out research into the toxicology of cyclamates. Without waiting for the publication of their findings, our Ministry of Agriculture, Fisheries and Food banned their use in food or drink from 1 January 1970.

New uses for sugar land and products
There may be some of you who are beginning to feel a little worried lest a wide and strongly supported campaign for the Abolition of Sugar Slavery might cause the Decline and Fall of the Empire of Mr Cube. Save your sobs, and consider some second thoughts. There are a number of ways in which his products could be usefully employed, and armies of workers re-deployed. These include the following:

1 Growing other crops on land released from sugar cane.
2 Making safe and fully soluble detergents.
3 Replacing wood as a source of newsprint.
4 Acting as a base for the production of protein.

5 Contributing, as molasses, up to 73 per cent of the dry matter in the diet of beef cattle.

6 Doing several odd jobs about the home.

1 In the Province of Natal in South Africa it has already been found that there is no need for despondency over crises in the sugar industry, as there are many crops that can again be grown in the cane belt. These only disappeared because their production and marketing compared unfavourably with sugar. Today, when the economic picture is very different, it has been discovered that tea, coffee, kenaf and cotton can all be developed on a substantial scale. This example could no doubt be followed in other cane-growing areas.

2 It is true that synthetic detergents have been improved in form recently so that they can now be broken down by bacteria in effluents, but they still cling to anything washed in them, and so are swallowed in food and drink, and they continue to overload inland waters with phosphates, turning many into fish cemeteries. So that it is encouraging to learn that the Tropical Products Institute in London has been working on turning sugar into detergents though there are still some difficulties over details. These detergents would not only be free from foam and phosphate troubles but would be digestible and if used 'to wash fruit and vegetables there would be no need to worry about traces of detergents left on the produce,' to quote the article in question.[12] This would seem to imply apparently that there certainly *is* need to worry about the present ones in use.

The Institute hoped that a whole range of industrial uses for sugar could arise out of its research, such as in lubricating, textile processing, the making of cosmetics and so on. This view is supported by independent work carried out in Nebraska.[13]

3 Newsprint made entirely from the waste from sugar-cane called bagasse was begun as a pioneer plant at Karad some 200 miles from Bombay some years ago,[14] and appears to foreshadow an expansion of newsprint production from cane-growing countries which could do much to reduce the drain on forests condemned to furnish material for this ever-greedier maw.

4 Yeast-producing factories in sugar belts now turn out 2000 lbs of protein from each five tons of sugar, the yield of one acre, compared with the yield of fifty lbs of protein per acre from beef cattle, according to John Laffin in his book *The Hunger to Come*.[15] This should basically reduce the world shortage of protein, could the food

be made acceptable to man. This seems highly probable, given the large number of nutritionally valueless or even harmful substances that have been made not only acceptable but attractive to eat or drink.

5 The potential of blackstrap molasses in animal feeds has been hampered in the past by the belief that it might be detrimental from its laxative effect, if given as more than 10–15 per cent of the diet. Recently, however, an important advance has been made in the feeding to beef cattle of diluted molasses, contributing up to 73 per cent of the dry matter in the diet, as a major source of energy for intensive animal production. It is expected that this will lead to a dramatic improvement in supplies of meat.[16]

6 Finally, there are a few household ways for using up any spare stocks. A lump of sugar to keep a silver teapot or picnic kettle 'sweet' is an old dodge known to most people, but here are two others recommended by Elizabeth Kendall which may be new to some of us.[17] To clean grimy hands, pour a little oil of any kind in the palms, add one teaspoon of castor sugar and work well until the sugar has melted. Dry on an old towel. Also, to keep larkspur from dropping and the leaves of chrysanthemums from wilting quickly, dissolve a teaspoon of sugar in warm water, cool and add to the vase contents. There is no need, either, to scrap as superfluous any icing sugar you may have in the cupboard. It can be usefully employed against ants when mixed with borax. (See Chapter 7.)

Thus, even the black cloud enshrouding sugar is found to possess a silver lining, and we may end, as Lincoln began, turning a foe in the wrong place into a friend in the right.

REFERENCES

1   *Ministry of Labour Gazette* HMSO (1966)
2   FREDERICKS, CARLTON and BAILEY, HERBERT. *Food Facts and Fallacies* (Here's Health Publ., 1966)
3   MATTICE, M. R., MA, DSC, *Bridges' Food and Beverage Analyses* (Henry Kimpton, 1950)
4   CLEAVE, C. T., MRCP, CHB (EDIN.), and CAMPBELL, G. D., MB, CHB (EDIN.) *Diabetes, Coronary Thrombosis and the Saccharine Diseases* (Wright, Bristol, 1965)
5   *New Scientist* (16 March 1967)
6   GERSTLEY, J. R. *et al. J. Pediat.*, 27, 521 (1945)
7   PRICE, WESTON, MS, DDS, FACD. *Nutrition and Physical Degeneration* published privately (1950)
8   *Safety of Artificial Sweeteners for Use in Foods*, Nut. Ac. Sci. Nat. Res. Council Publ. 386 (1955)

9   CONSUMER REPORTS (October 1964)
10   THOMPSON, M. M. *et al. Am. J. Clin. Nut.*, 7, 80 (1959)
11   BAKER, H. *et al. Nature*, 191, 78 (1961)
12   *New Scientist* (16 October 1961)
13   *Ibid.* (27 October 1966)
14   *South African Industrial Chemist* (June 1961)
15   LAFFIN, JOHN. *The Hunger to Come* (Abelard Schuman, 1966)
16   ORESTON, T. R. *et al. Rev. Cubana Cienc. Agric.*, Vol. 1 (1967)
17   KENDALL, ELIZABETH. *House into Home* (Aldin. Publ., 1966)

10

Fatness or Fitness?

'A Century ago it was considered normal for Man to be
obese, but we have learned it isn't normal.'
DR EWAN CAMERON

Even if education and example succeed in abolishing sugar
addiction, we still face the fact of widespread addiction to food
which is 'one of the leading health hazards of modern urban societies',
in the opinion of Dr William Phillips.

A recent mass observation survey found that one in every ten
adults is trying to slim at this moment—one in three if women only
are considered—but 45 per cent gave up after one year and only 3
per cent struggled on to final victory. In America the picture is even
worse with seventy-nine million overweight people, according to
The Overweight Society by Peter Wyden.[1] There, 'Mr Big' of Philadelphia holds the World Weight record with 644 lbs (46 stone), won
on pie, ice cream, cake mixes and 'french fried' in the home country
of refined carbohydrates.

Britain lags behind, but today, our Fatties begin building their
bulges even before birth, for leading authorities consider anything
over 8 lbs at birth undesirable. There are medical officers of health
who believe that baby shows should be abolished, because they put a
premium on the bigger baby and so encourage mothers to overfeed
their infants. It seems probable that this error of judgement may also
stem from the universal practice at welfare clinics of weighing infants,
and appearing to give better 'marks' for greater gains every week.
Though, of course, a steady weight gain is a good indication that
development is going well and everyone wants a bonny not a bony
baby. While early plumpness spells contentment, a fat infant is a
sluggish one, and laying the foundation for an obese and slothful
schoolchild.

How many parents are aware that obesity is a serious defect which
should not be allowed to occur? Where have we slipped off the dotted

line that keeps us in nutritional balance? Why are so many of us almost totally innocent of the importance of this balance? How is it that we tolerate the fact that between 20 and 30 per cent of the middle-aged in civilized countries are to be considered obese? Finally, why is it only common knowledge with insurance companies and not all of us that, as one physician has put it, 'every fat person is signing his own death warrant'?

The causes of obesity
We have to be quite certain of one thing, about which many people seem very uncertain, i.e. the causes of obesity. 'Too few patients appreciate that the cause of obesity is over-eating, and many are not convinced that their obesity is related to their food intake,' says Dr R. M. Harden of Glasgow. The first thing, then, is to accept the fact that overeating leads to overweight, and that only reduced eating can lead to reduced weight. Aiding and abetting overeating are lazy limbs in every age group—lying unmoved in a pram, sitting in a car, taking part only in spectator sports, and generally making as little effort as possible throughout the day. Aware of these basic causes, we can resolve to cope, both for those for whom we are responsible, and for ourselves.

Dr Robert Kemp warned in an issue of the *Practitioner* early in 1967 that we are on the way to becoming a nation of 'fatties'. He stated that there are more fat children than ever before, which he attributes to an excessive consumption of white bread, sugar, sweets and potatoes. This indictment of sweets should surprise no one who has watched children rushing out of school to flock to confectioners, sucking sweets at all hours, and piling sugar on foods which are already sweetened. I venture to disagree, though, about putting blame on potatoes—except as crisps of course, when their calories are doubled. Organically grown and properly home-cooked potatoes contain sufficient vitamins to convert them into the energy so freely expended by the young; and there were no tubby Irish peasants in the days when they lived largely on milk, potatoes and salt.

The disadvantage of obesity
Activity of any sort spends energy, and the extra energy entailed in breaking down or metabolizing additional body fat may severely overtax the lungs and heart, while if the heart is already diseased even a minor degree of obesity may lead to heart failure. Excess

weight throws extra work on the body-bearing joints of hip, knee and ankle, and undue strain on all the ligaments concerned, leading to pain of varying severity. The insulating effect of fat may cause great discomfort in hot weather or in doing any form of physical labour, and increased vital statistics may be responsible for difficulty in buying any ready-made clothes that are not vastly unbecoming.

Starting at the beginning
1 Since all body-building begins in the womb, every pregnant person should aim at an ordinary, not an outsize, baby, taking care not to eat for more than two, and choosing foods and drinks in accordance with the best nutritional advice. And, of course, care should be taken to ensure adequate daily exercise. Incidentally, it seems probable that having big babies may lead to diabetes in the mother. From a follow-up carried out at the General Hospital, Birmingham, of sixty-one mothers, thirteen years after they had produced infants weighing over ten and a half lbs at birth, it was found that half were already diabetic and it was estimated that at least half of the rest would become so in the next ten years.[2]

2 The mother of a baby content to lie still and merely stare indefinitely, thus earning a reputation for being 'such a good boy/girl', should not be commended. Healthy unbulging babies display vigour and movement as soon as they are allowed to lie, free of trappings, on their tummy. This should begin during the first month of life, for soon attempts to wriggle will follow and progress until he can move about and starts to crawl. It has been found that crawling is an invaluable exercise, helping to develop brain as well as body. So at this stage it is a mistake to restrict a child to a playpen; he needs to be physically free to use all his senses which are his five ways of learning about the world and to use that co-ordination of foot, hand and eye which are encouraged by the act of crawling. Further, the sides of a pen tend to make him cling on and stand before he is ready for this and cut short the valuable crawling stage. In a warm room, with bare feet so that he learns the use of his toes, and with all potentially dangerous objects out of reach, energies can be fully expended and powers developed before any walking is attempted.

3 The fat schoolchild is so often the butt of his companions that mere common kindness dictates that he should be helped to see the advantages of reducing his weight and encouraged to become more

active, even if this only means being sent on more errands for mother rather than sitting in front of a TV screen, and given apples to nibble rather than toffee. The fat child may not develop varicose veins or heart trouble for many decades; he may indeed be well over fifty before he pays the price for early overweight, but pay he must sooner or later.

4 The slothful and too often spotty adolescent can usually be enticed by reasons of vanity into eating at least fewer sugar products, and perhaps persuaded to substitute such excellent exercise as cycling, swimming and dancing for merely sitting about in cafés and watching TV, or other people engaging in sports.

5 For sedentary workers a splendid lead was given in 1966 by the Maryland State Government which permitted all its men and women employees to spend ten minutes a day during office time at a physical fitness break in an effort, approved by their Board of Public Works, to help 'take off the fat'. A press report shows that this example has already been followed in Brussels. How long before our own traditional tea break is preceded by PT for all?

The sex angle

While it is still true that inside every fat man there is a thin one struggling to get out, this also applies to fat women, of whom there are many more. At the Royal Hospital for Sick Children, Glasgow, Dr J. Oman Craig has reported that females are the fat sex, and Mr Phillip Lebon, the consultant who founded the Obesity Association, has estimated that a mere 18 per cent of men are overweight as compared with 25 per cent of women. For students in America aspiring to universities there is a higher rejection rate for fat men than thin applicants of roughly equal intelligence, according to a survey in 1966 by the Harvard University School of Public Health. This discrimination applies in a greater degree to overweight girls since clothing styles are said to make feminine obesity more apparent.[3]

From the USA also comes the demolition of the myth of the 'jolly fat girl'. Psychiatrists at the Children's Hospital, Washington, studying obese teenage girls and normal weight contemporaries, have reported that this jollity is merely a façade beneath which she is likely to be depressed and anxious, while denying the problems associated with her obesity. They consider that these cases need close supervision and diet control from parents and doctor, and this advice would seem to apply to anyone who is immensely fat but minutely resolute.

Preliminary precautions
1 Don't diet, then indulge. This makes the body weight rocket up and down, upsets the cholesterol balance, tending to 'fur up' the arteries, and lead to heart trouble.

2 Don't fall for so-called slimming foods. These don't exist except in advertisements. *Fattening foods do*, and these must be learned by heart and avoided.

3 Don't use any form of synthetic sweetener. These are under suspicion as carcinogens, rapidly destroy vitamin C and can damage the liver. A leading article in the *Lancet* (15 January 1966) can be summarized as follows. Safety decisions are not permanent in connection with the permitted use of cyclamates (acids, sodium and calcium salts) as synthetic sweeteners. In the USA these have not been used in food since 1950. Here their use was sanctioned by the Ministry of Health (Soft Drink Regulations 1964 S.I. 1964/760), but the Minister of Agriculture, Fisheries and Food announced on 23 October 1969 that in the light of information received from the USA it was felt that there 'cannot be certainty about the safety of cyclamates without further information'. Until additional research has been carried out, therefore, it has been decided that cyclamates should not be added to food or drink of any kind including sweetening preparations.

4 Don't try to reduce appetite by taking strong coffee, cocoa or tea as they can cause insomnia, and damage the liver.

5 Don't turn to smoking as an appetite reducer, since this habit harms the heart which is already under strain as the result of excess poundage.

6 Don't cut down meals to one or two daily, for infrequent meals swamp the body's labour force of enzymes, which retaliate by storing what they are unable to cope with as fat.

7 Don't go without breakfast, causing a fall in blood sugar which produces a hunger for the chocolate bars and chocolate biscuits at morning tea break. Your breakfast can be protein rich and non-fattening; at work or school only fattening carbohydrates will be available easily.

8 Don't underestimate the value of dodging temptation in the form of a favourite fattener. Ask yourself if it is worthwhile to seek

out those chocolates or whatever, when you have a few permitted peanuts, almonds or a knob of cheese ready to hand.

9 Don't protest that you only eat like a bird, remembering the voracious vulture.

10 Don't forget that unless fat is burned efficiently in working off energy (and this requires almost every nutrient and especially vitamin B_6), it cannot be budged from unwanted places. Make full use of brewer's yeast, the best source of vitamin B complex.

11 Don't waste money on firmer foundations which only re-distribute bulges, nor on so-called 'slimming garments' which merely make one lose weight from heavy sweating, quickly replaced by drinking and eating.

12 Don't overlook the fact that self-esteem, when earned by self-discipline, is a good thing, since it is an aid to esteeming others. So give yourself frequent pats on the back for what you are achieving.

A cool look at slimming methods

It is quite mistaken to suppose anyone trying to slim must take appetite-reducing pills or go hungry most of the time. Such pills are now recognized as dangerous and possibly addictive, and with a little basic knowledge about which foods are better value than others the would-be slimmer can feel satisfied physically and psychologically. It also pays to cultivate incredulity about claims for specially pre-pared foods, since few of these would support even a bacterium. Better nutrients, not worse, are required by the obese.

Few fatties have the insight or the honesty of that ponderous rogue elephant Orson Welles, who admitted in a radio interview to the vice of gluttony, commenting wryly, 'Most vices are secret, but gluttony shows. And by it we make a mess of ourselves.' Yet the first step towards reducing weight must be to admit the necessity of reducing.

Facing up to fattening foods

'All flesh is grass,' said the Psalmist. For the would-be slimmer this could be amended to 'All unwanted flesh is the product of a giant grass (the sugar cane) or the secret sugars that ape it.' A single helping of sweetened breakfast cereal or one with every flake coated with sugar, white bread and jam, biscuits, an ice, pastry, pudding, tinned fruit, jelly or cake, contributes the equivalent of two to three table-spoons of white sugar, and may add up to as much as one to two cupfuls in the day consumed by someone who really believes that he or she has most righteously 'not eaten any sugar at all'.

Rodale's story of the young diabetic sailor who was wrecked on a Pacific island shows that drastic pruning of all possible sources of such harmful sugars can almost work miracles. One would have thought he would have been in a bad way, having lost his insulin, but when he was rescued some weeks later he was no longer diabetic. He had been forced to live on nothing but fish and fruit, and had had no access to any of the 'secret sugars' or sugar.

One wishes that a lengthy stay on a desert island could have been arranged for one of the best-loved fat men in our history, since it would probably not only have relieved him of the burden of his unwieldy weight, but also of the 'vile melancholy' to which he was a frequent prey, as Boswell so sadly recalls. Dr Samuel Johnson began as a lean and lanky young man. There can be little doubt that he owed many of his later physical infirmities to his habit, on sitting down to table, of plunging his hands at once in the common sugar bowl—until Mrs Thrale ordered the bowl to be taken away—and of course he ate hugely as well. Eating more than very minor amounts of white sugar, or indeed any similarly emasculated starchy food which is converted in the body into pyruvic acid or sucrose, means that a series of surpluses arise which house themselves in such vacant sites as the lower cheeks and chin, the abdominal muscles and the back of the neck. Furthermore, this leaves neither room nor appetite for proteins, and this imbalance according to Professor Duddington, the fungus expert, causes even yeasts, like humans, to accumulate deposits of fat in their cells.[4]

Yeasts are forced to feed on what they are given. Adult humans (except of course those in practically every kind of institution, either as workers or patients) are not so forced. It has always been man's proud boast that he has chosen freedom. In fact it appears that Freedom of Choice in Food should indeed be added to the Four Freedoms established by Roosevelt. As Professor Sherman has written, 'It is now clear, for those who will study the evidence, that even in the everyday choice of food we are dealing with values that are above price for the health, efficiency, duration and dignity of human life.'

General principles

Before embarking on any reducing programme it is important to realize that what matters is not entirely the amount of food eaten, but whether it contains the factors required to convert fat into energy. These factors are *not* present in any refined flour, cereal or sugar products, nor in hydrogenated fats (liquid oils made solid by adding water), whether of animal or vegetable origin, but they *are* present in wholemeal flour and cereals, molasses and vegetable oils. In fact it has been found that patients asked merely to substitute oil for solid fats and to limit sugars and starches, felt so well satisfied because the oil decreased their hunger (since it is slow in digestion and speeds up the burning of the lumps of saturated body fat) that they were content with far fewer calories, and all lost weight. Since protein readily satisfies hunger, supplies energy-producing enzymes, and helps the liver to produce the enzymes necessary to inactivate insulin, it also prevents that hollow feeling and craving for sweet foods that hits one when the blood sugar falls. So protein should be eaten generously. In fact, the aim should be to concentrate on worthwhile foods which increase energy production, and discard all others, while plenty of green leaf vegetables and fresh fruit should be eaten for their mineral and vitamin value.

Counting proteins not calories
A health-building as well as weight-reducing daily programme must contain a minimum of about sixty grams of protein for a woman and eighty for a man. Containing only natural fats and only complete proteins are butter, milk, fresh and powdered skim milk (for adding to soups, mayonnaise, etc.), wheat germ, soya flour (for adding to wholemeal bread, gravies, etc.) and brewer's yeast. Liver, heart, kidney, eggs, cabbage, skim milk, cheese and fish, are very low in solid fats.

Fish for the figure
Fish still feed on the plankton of sea pastures which are never depleted of minerals as are so many soil pastures today, and they are perhaps the best source of protein for non-vegetarians. They are also less expensive, contain fewer calories than an equivalent helping of meat, and are rich in poly-unsaturated fats.* Beware of fish fried in batter—the last word in fat-producing and objectionable factors—consisting of white flour cooked in re-heated saturated (i.e. solid)

* Liquid vegetable and fish oils essential for the utilization of saturated (solid) fats such as butter, meat fats, etc. Experts consider them preventative of abnormal fat deposits in arteries, a condition called 'atherosclerosis'.

fats which destroy part of the vitamin A activity of other food eaten at the same time.

Boiled fish, that horror of boarding school Fridays, is a desecration of a food which can be made inviting by grilling, baking, casseroling, or simmering in milk with onions, tomatoes, herbs, curry powder, cheese, mushrooms, egg, either singly, or combined according to taste. Nor should the fish eaten begin and end with cod. It should include halibut, turbot, fresh haddock, skate (especially the tail sold as Dutch eel), ling and whiting, to name only a few. Also all fatty varieties such as herrings and mackerel, well grilled until the fat has been melted out and the bones made crisp enough to eat as a source of calcium. Alternatively, a teaspoon of salt can be sprinkled in the pan before heating it thoroughly, then poured off and the well-dried fish tossed until it is brown and crisp. A simple sauce can consist of finely chopped parsley in peanut, or sunflower seed oil (better value than olive), rather than butter, or mayonnaise (home-made) if the fish is to be eaten cold with a salad.

It is a pity that prawns, shrimps, scallops, etc. are so expensive for they are extra good value nutritionally and add variety. Finally, in favour of fish, comes the thyroid-feeding iodine it supplies—to be found in iodized salt by the non-flesh eater. This enables the body to raise its basal metabolic rate, causing all foods to be utilized more rapidly and completely, leaving no surplus to accumulate as rolls of fat.

Getting familiar with fats
Anyone who can pinch one inch of fat between thumb and finger just above their waistline, on the upper arm, or just above their lowest rib, not only qualifies as obese, but has learned that body fat in the human is saturated or solid fat. To burn this up it is necessary to supply the essential fatty acids (EFAs) found in liquid vegetable, nut, and fish oils, at the rate of not more than two tablespoons daily. This should be spread over the day since only a limited amount can be coped with at a time and any surplus is liable to be stored as flabby fat. Adelle Davis[5] suggests taking these necessary oils six times daily at the equivalent rate of one teaspoon each in the form of ten large peanuts, one walnut, one teaspoon mayonnaise, two teaspoons dried sunflower seeds or non-hydrogenated peanut-butter, while any vegetable can be served with oil instead of butter, and potato mashed with a little warm milk and a similar addition.

Incidentally, it is better to exclude brazil and cashew nuts, which happen to be rich in saturated fats. Cooking entirely with oil, carefully measured not to exceed the two tablespoons per day, not only cuts out undesirable solid fats and adds beneficial ones, but helps to make reducing easier, because of the high satiety value of fats. A satisfied stomach is far less likely to crave forbidden foods than a hungry one. On no account should liquid paraffin be used, although it adds no calories, since it steals the fat soluble vitamins, A, D, E and K.

Firm girdles or firmer muscles?
While foundation garments can boost morale they merely redistribute flesh or fat, and tend to increase the flabbiness of the natural girdle of abdominal muscles which exercise alone can strengthen and restore to firmness. Here are some very simple ways in which muscles and skin can be tightened up, as weight is lost. Best done nude, or in a bathing suit.

1 Stand upright with the feet astride, with the arms hanging loosely at the side. Breathe *out* through the mouth with a hissing sound and try to touch the ground with the outstretched finger tips without bending the knees. Now rotate the palms outwards and breathe *in* through the nose, while lifting up to the starting position. Repeat three to six times.

2 Lying down, draw up both feet on the floor until the knees are at a right angle, then breathe *out* with the same hissing breath drawing up the right knee as far as possible towards the face. Lower again to starting position while breathing *in* through the nose. Pause. Repeat with left knee. Repeat three to six times.

3 Lying, with knees still at right angles breathe *out*, then breathe *in* lifting the buttocks and lower ribs clear, hold for a few seconds, then lower to starting position while breathing *out*. Repeat three to six times.

4 Lying flat with hands at the side and feet together, draw up the right leg at the hip without bending the knee while breathing *out*, sliding the left hand down the side of the leg. Draw back hand and foot to starting position while breathing *in*. Repeat with left leg and arm. Repeat three to six times.

When you can do these exercises perfectly, increase by doing one more every time, until you reach twelve.

N.B. The tone of the abdominal muscles can be greatly improved if when sitting, the buttocks are pushed back as far as possible into the seat, the head and shoulders held erect above this base, and the abdominal muscles are pulled in strongly, so pressing the spine against the back of the seat. This can be practised quite unperceived in bus or car, etc., and is very useful.

Take some outdoor exercise every day. This can be walking, bicycling, gardening, or what you will. If you cannot get out, then walk up and down the stairs as often as possible until you get breathless. You will find the number of times will increase gradually. Never take vigorous exercise or play games for at least an hour after a meal.

A TV diet

A diet sheet under the above title approved by the BMA was sent out free to applicants in 1967. Though a move in the right direction it appears far too permissive over certain items. For example:

1 Blancmange and other cornflour and white flour products.
2 Unlimited tea and coffee.
3 Low calorie soft drinks, under suspicion for their content of cyclamate which is now banned in this country.

The psychology of eating

Research so far has concentrated on the physiology of eating Experiments by a professor of psychology at Columbia University[6] suggest that the study of the psychology of eating might throw further light on the problem of obesity, though it seems uncertain whether this would assist in the practical treatment of obesity with which most of us who are overweight are concerned.

Obviously we can't expect to live as if fattening up ourselves for the livestock market, and yet live up to our highest potential. The aim in feeding livestock is to make them grow fast and large, to bring in a fat profit when slaughtered. For ourselves, what is the aim? Could it be to grow into balanced beings, with a capacity to attain physical, mental and spiritual vigour and to maintain this to the end of the road, whenever that may be?

REFERENCES

1   WYDEN, PETER. *The Overweight Society* (Evans, 1966)
2   *Lancet*, 7189, 1250
3   HARVARD UNIVERSITY SCHOOL OF PUBLIC HEALTH (1966)
4   DUDDINGTON, C. L. *Micro-organisms as Allies* (Faber, 1961)

5   DAVIS, ADELLE. *Let's Get Well* (George Allen and Unwin, 1966)
6   SCHLACHTER S. *Science* (1 September 1968)

RECOMMENDED READING FOR SLIMMERS

YUDKIN, PROFESSOR JOHN. *The Complete Slimmer* (MacGibbon and Kee, 1964) This is very helpful and serious, yet highly amusing.

11

Food Defences against Cancer

'From now on medical science should be directed towards research into the various factors involved in natural immunity.'

DR ALEXIS CARREL

People are at least as important as poultry. Pressure of public opinion led to the Brambell Report with the aim of improving living conditions for animals. Why do we submit without adequate protest to polluted living conditions for ourselves? Meanwhile, and until the ideal dawn of *no pollution, no carcinogens,* begins to glimmer in the future, sound and informed nutrition can help to build and fortify the natural defensive systems of the body to repulse its many enemies, especially the condition known to most of us as cancer.

Few can be unaware that although diseases such as smallpox have been driven back by modern man, cancer has advanced to an alarming degree among all sorts and conditions of men, women and children. Once an affliction mostly confined to the elderly, cancer now attacks at any time of life, and even before birth. What is being done to teach people how they can protect themselves and their families? What are the weapons of defence recommended by preventive medicine?

The year 1967 saw the publication of *The Prevention of Cancer* (Butterworths) edited by Ronald W. Raven, OBE, TD, FRCS, and Francis J. C. Roe, DM, DSc, MCPath., with contributions by fifty eminent authorities in the field of cancer. Undoubtedly this is a monument to devoted work, but with all due deference, it seems in spite of its vast bulk to have three important omissions in so far as the general public is concerned.

1 There is no report by a molecular biologist, a physiologist or a nutritionist, in spite of reference to the possibility that the proliferation of abnormal cells derived from normal cells in which cancer usually begins, may arise from one single cell, with the relevance of

this fact for the study of structure, function and nutrition of normal cells.

2 Avowedly this book is 'intended not only for the medical profession but for all interested or involved in the problems of human wealth and welfare'. Surely this should include us all. Yet how many are equipped mentally or semantically to understand the scientific and medical terms in which it is couched?

3 The further aim is to 'outline *practical* measures which on present knowledge can be taken to prevent the disease'. We search in vain for this promised outline. There are lists of potential carcinogens derived from foods due to cooking practices, processing and preservation, contamination by man-made chemicals such as insecticides, detergents, antibiotics and metals, chemical additives such as dyes and flavouring and sterilization by irradiation. Attention is drawn to the toxicity of cosmetic, toilet and pharmaceutical preparations, X-rays for diagnosis or therapy, trauma and viruses. There is advice to avoid smoking, betel or tobacco chewing, taking snuff, exposure to noxious fumes, eating raw fish, etc. Dietary excesses, dietary imbalances, liver damage and the importance of a balanced diet for the prevention of gastric cancer are all mentioned, including the suggestion that since man is the only animal to suffer from cancer of the rectum, a study should be made of the effects of cooking. These are guidelines. Where is the required manual of instruction?

There have been many previous warnings from responsible quarters that man should avoid or banish these well-documented hazards. But how is this to be done? What are the 'practical measures' which can be taken to prevent the disease? Surely this means those protective measures which can be carried out in any home? Details of these are conspicuously lacking anywhere in this volume.

We can no longer pretend that cancer is solely a matter for the experts. It concerns us all, here and now. We are all at risk. Since no one up to the present appears to have given a simple account of such protective measures as are already known and can be used by anyone responsible enough to take the trouble, there follows, with references to first-hand expert opinions and findings, an outline of what has been culled from many sources and mulled over for years, in the hope that this may be helpful to every housewife and to others. There is indeed much we can do to protect and prevent. We can each start today in our home, before carrying the work out into the wider field of the world.

Protective measures against cancer

Cancer is no new disease. It probably reaches back to the first use of fire, and cases are recorded in the Ebers papyrus dated 1500 BC. Among the carcinogens present among the early Egyptians must have been benzanthracenes, occurring when foods are roasted at high temperatures, carbon monoxide from fuel combustion and a predisposing factor in a deficiency of vitamin B complex owing to leaching by irrigation. These are still present, but technological man has increased their range and variety so enormously that there are today over one thousand man-made carcinogens, unknown fifty years ago, to be found in food and drink alone. How much longer shall we continue to disregard these essential facts of life?

The most disturbing aspect of cancer is that it has widened its jaws to engulf not only the elderly, as in former centuries, but also infants and children, so that in Britain it is second only to accidents as the commonest cause of death among children aged one to fifteen years,[1] and in the USA there were 500,000 deaths of infants due to cancer in 1958, although such deaths had been very rare in the 1930s.[2] Why is this?

The answer is not certain, but an eminent authority, Dr W. C. Hueper of the National Cancer Institute of the USA, has suggested that this may be related to carcinogens to which the mother has been exposed in pregnancy which have passed through the placental barrier to act on her unborn child.[3]

Until recent years cancer had the status of a four letter word. Today, it can be as freely referred to as say, aberrant sex for, thanks to the commonsense approach of Richard Dimbleby and other victims, a subject of great public and private significance can now be openly discussed. But publicity is not enough. The smoke screen of silence has been pierced. We have had the revolt so now let us turn it into a revolution. We must bombard the authorities and ourselves with questions demanding an answer in no uncertain voice.

Admittedly, it is much easier to focus attention on clean hands—important though these are—than on the ubiquitous carcinogens present in the food being handled. But why has no publicity been given to the statement by the American Association for the Advancement of Science that when any substance is found to be carcinogenic, many scientists consider its use in food to be unsafe, because this property of carcinogenicity is unique, and a threshold (safe) dose has not been established?[4]

A society called CETEX was formed some years before the assaults on the uninhabited moon, concerned with protecting the world against Contamination by Extra-Terrestrial Experiment. Why is there no such society dedicated to protecting the enormously in-habited earth from our thousands of contaminating and man-made carcinogens?

Clearly, it is up to each one of us as individuals to cope as best we can. This requires relevant knowledge too often lacking or ignored. To deny today the link between cancer of the lung and cigarettes shows either a vested interest in tobacco sales, or a misguided im-itation of Nelson with the telescope to his blind eye. However, tobacco is in no way obligatory. We need not smoke, but we must all eat and drink.

We humans have fitted Nancy Mitford's description of a broiler for too long: 'The kind of creature you keep in the dark, and feed on injections.' It is high time that there was a national campaign aimed at making known the recognized carcinogens in food and fluids, and how to protect ourselves against them.

The British Empire Cancer Campaign and the Imperial Cancer Relief Fund finance research into the causes, nature and treatment of cancer, and the National Society for Cancer Relief issues a leaflet from its information centre whose terms of reference include, 'To spread health education, and to collate and distribute information on cancer and health education free of cost to the public'. An excellent aim, but careful reading of the leaflet reveals absolutely no mention of protective factors.

In 1966, a visiting American professor's widely reported statement that the British were wasting millions on cancer research, aroused great controversy. Many of us would agree that many of these millions are indeed misdirected and should be spent on the en-lightenment of the public about known carcinogens, and how to avoid or at least counteract them, since these are known in some degree. He was also reported as wanting a summit conference of research experts but this had already taken place in Rome in 1956, when the conclusion reached by the forty-two experts from the twenty-one countries represented was 'The urgent necessity for international collaboration for the protection of mankind against chemical additives'. Furthermore, they authorized a sub-committee to write a report on the hidden perils of chemical additives in food. Why was this not proclaimed by the Press throughout the world? John Lear,

American Correspondent of the *New Scientist*, soon found out why. He published the findings of the committee in full in the US *Saturday Review*. Then, to quote his own words, 'The enraged howls of the chemical advertisers scared the newspapers off the story, but it was too late to prevent the one publication of the text of the report itself from selling out completely.' A subsequent word-of-mouth campaign among American consumers finally induced Congress to pass a law setting strict control on all food additives.

'*Methods of protection against cancer* must henceforth occupy first place in the struggle against cancer,' announced the great cancer specialist Bauer to his colleagues in Germany at the Cancer Congress in 1954.[5] Why have these protective methods never been passed on to the public by the appropriate authorities?

Facing the enemy

A necessary basis for defence or attack is to know something of the essential nature of the enemy. Here is a recent definition by Dr Peter Stubbs: 'Cancer is not a single disease, but a large group all characterized by the fact that the cells making up one or several parts of an organism grow in an uncontrolled fashion. There are several theories as to why this happens, but there is little doubt that something has happened to the cell's genetic material known as DNA.'*[6]

Basically, people split into two groups when faced with any great problem. The first looks away or asks, 'What are *they* going to do about it?' The second considers, 'What are *we* going to do?', and looks about for clues. Where in cancer prevention does the real responsibility lie? Surely with all of us in the second group, since it is we who can decide what we shall breathe, eat and drink in our homes, and what we shall ban.

It has been calculated that by cutting out only the outdoor environmental carcinogens that surround us 70 per cent of cancer could be prevented, but this would entail spending time, trouble and thousands of millions on getting rid first of the air pollution through smoke, exhaust fumes and so on which are a blight in every atmosphere except those remote from man and his miasmas. How many are

---

* It is encouraging to note that Professor John D. Watson, joint winner of a Nobel prize for elucidating the structure of the DNA molecule, is now studying, as Director of the Cold Harbour Laboratory of Quantitive Biology, the biochemical and molecular events that lead to cancer.[7]

prepared to treat this as a priority and take action? The Clean Air Act is a mere straw in the wind so far. It is going to take the mightiest hurricane man ever knew to sweep away the monarchy of the internal combustion engine, which now rules and pollutes the roads, and treats the attempted development of a non-polluting electric engine as high treason, and it will take a far more clear-sighted decade than our own to allow human lives to take precedence over human locomotion.

What the individual can do
We are not, as individuals, able to control the atmosphere outside our walls, but it is certainly up to us to reduce our daily intake of polluted air indoors by the methods suggested in earlier chapters.

Next, we can and should do all we can to avoid the potential carcinogens condemned alike by the Rome experts and the authors of *The Prevention of Cancer*, i.e. the dyes, flavourings, sweeteners, bleaches, antioxidants and preservatives to be found in commercial jams, jellies, ices, sweets, cakes, biscuits, custard powders, mixes, margarines, bottled drinks, tinned vegetables, oil and fat substitutes, mineral oils, liquid paraffin especially, anti-sprouting agents on potatoes and onions, antibiotics and hormones used for fattening poultry and cattle. For, according to the cancer specialist, Dr W. C. Hueper, 'It is wise to eliminate from human food any substance which has been found to cause cancer in any animal by any route of administration.'[8]

What of the equally condemned detergents and pesticide residues present in most foods and all waters today? However, we may try, we cannot now avoid these. There was an acid comment made after the death of Rachel Carson by a woman inclined to pooh-pooh *Silent Spring*: 'Surely she knew enough to avoid carcinogens?' The point is that even anyone so well-informed could not possibly avoid them in the chemical-ridden USA any more than we can in Britain today. It seems probable that she was as unaware as most of us of the means for protection against what have become inevitable hazards on every hand. What does this protection consist of?

No panaceas, but no need to feel powerless
It must be emphasized that in this field, as in all others, there are *no*

panaceas. There are, however, simple protective factors we can all invoke and provide, once we have the know-how.

Our first action must be to banish fear. This not only chases out happiness, but upsets the adrenal glands, two of our stoutest allies in any struggle. Sir Heneage Ogilvy, the eminent physician, asked years ago, 'What is the force which keeps it [cancer] at bay in the great majority of us?' and his own reply was, 'The happy man never gets cancer.' Be that as it may, we can all derive a degree of comfort from the knowledge that we are doing all we can to protect our households from this enemy.

The nature of this protection was indicated as long ago as 1941 by Professor Maisin of the Cancer Institute, Louvain, when he wrote, 'In certain vegetables and foodstuffs there are one or two factors which are active in the prophylaxis [prevention of, or protection against] cancer caused by the azo dyes and hydrocarbons which are the dangers with which we are now concerned.'[9] This statement was confirmed eight years later by the great German cancer specialist Bauer (a surgeon, be it noted, not a nutritionist), in the words, 'We are justified in concluding that nutrition, whatever its nature, can favour cancer, or on the other hand protect against it',[10] and at the Cancer Congress in Germany in 1954 he confessed that he placed his last hope in protective measures against cancer.[11]

Bauer's major work, *Das Krebsproblem* (*The Cancer Problem*), published in 1949 and still one of the most complete encyclopedias on the subject, has this to say: 'The fact that the carcinogenic influence of azo dyes cannot be exerted if the ration contains sufficient *riboflavin* is a discovery of fundamental importance for our methods of defence against cancer. It shows, in effect, that *we need no longer be exposed to the danger of carcinogenic action if we see to it that our diet is not deficient in a fundamental vitamin.*

'No one can believe that this is a unique and exceptional case. On the contrary, this example justifies *the conclusion that the diet, whatever its nature, can favour cancer, if, for a long period of time, it is lacking in certain essential substances.*'

These were encouraging words indeed, even in those days of far fewer cases, but as André Voisin comments, 'Unfortunately, they do not seem to have found much echo.'[12] At least, not among the bodies concerned with cancer research. These continue to pile up knowledge of causes, although over one thousand carcinogens are known to be in common use in our foods today, while methods of protection remain unheeded and unpublicized.

The importance of riboflavin (vitamin B$_2$)

The basis for the belief categorically stated above was a series of extremely important rat experiments carried out originally in Japan from 1932 to 1940, and repeated in Britain and the USA. The final conclusion reached was that the development of cancer of the liver due to azo dyes depends on the nature of the cereal portion of the ration and the treatment it has received, and that *whole* wheat has a remarkable capacity for preventing the cancer-causing action of these artificial dyes on the liver, though the way in which it works was not entirely clear. Later it was found that the protective factor present in whole wheat consists of that part of the water-soluble vitamin B complex known as riboflavin (B$_2$).[13]

What is riboflavin, and where else but in the whole wheat is it to be found? Being essential to every living cell it was once called the Royal vitamin, and it is present in varying degrees in all plants and animals. Since it is so widely distributed in nature, one would think that there could be no shortage in the diet of any but the under-privileged. This is definitely not so. In fact, it is the most universal of the vitamin deficiencies[14] and not at all infrequent, according to a well-known American authority, among people of professional standing.[15] This is due to the fact that it is unstable, and can be so easily destroyed or reduced by kitchen or other treatments, such as milling. Here an extraction rate of 85 per cent or over is necessary for the preservation of the riboflavin content of the wheat, and white flour has an extraction rate of 70 per cent only.[16]

Some sources of riboflavin[17]

Excellent	Good	Fair	Poor	None
Brewer's yeast	Wheat germ	Dates	Fruits	Sugar
Liver	Soya flour	Eggs	Oils	
Kidney	Tuna fish	Spinach	Potatoes	
Yogurt	Cheese	Almonds	Brown rice	
	Peanuts			
	Fresh milk			
	Whole dried lentils			

Ordinary daily requirements of humans[18]

Man		Woman		Child	
Sedentary	⎰1·6 mg	Sedentary	⎰1·5 mg	Under 1 year	⎰0·5 mg
to	⎱	to	⎱	to	⎱
very active	2·6 mg	very active	2·2 mg	10–12 years	1·5 mg
	Boy			*Girl*	
	13–15 years	⎰1·9 mg		13–15 years	⎰1·6 mg
	to	⎱		to	⎱
	16–20 years	2·1 mg		16–20 years	1·5 mg

Requirements increased by:
Chronic alcoholism,[19] an increase of fat in the diet,[20] pregnancy and lactation,[21] oily skin and hair,[22] accidents, surgery and burns.[23]

Robbers of riboflavin
Riboflavin is destroyed or much reduced in the kitchen by soaking and boiling vegetables and throwing away the water,[24] exposure to light in cooking or storage (transparent milk bottles ensuring that a great deal of the riboflavin content is lost),[25] antibiotics,[26] (often consumed unwittingly through veterinary treatments of stock), antacids, such as soda in cooking or as used in indigestion mixtures or tablets,[27] long-continued therapeutic diets[28] and those with a high fat content.[29]

A simple way of obtaining more riboflavin (and also vitamin C) is to sprout grains or beans, a custom throughout the East.[30] Doris Grant in *Housewives Beware* (Faber & Faber, 1958) describes the following method: 'Place six tablespoons of washed whole wheat in a wide-mouthed bottling jar, cover with four times as much lukewarm water and leave to soak overnight. Next morning, pour off the water, cover the jar with a piece of butter-muslin kept in place by a rubber band. Soak the wheat for a minute or so three times a day with lukewarm water, turning the jar upside down to drain. Do not allow the wheat to become chilled or the growth will be retarded and the wheat will become musty. Allow the sprouts to grow till they are about the length of the seed, but they are ready to use as soon as the sprouts are visible. They take about three days to germinate, and can then be stored in a closed jar in a refrigerator for three to four days. They can be used as a breakfast dish chopped up with top milk and honey, or added to soups, stews, sandwiches, salads and in making bread.'

During pregnancy the child draws heavily on the mother's reserve of riboflavin and her need becomes greater too, which may cause heartburn at about the fifth month.[31] Taking indigestion mixtures *reduces* her intake of riboflavin, while masking the effect. More, not less, riboflavin is necessary. Eating sprouted wheat is a cheap way of building up this deficiency. Under normal conditions there may be a certain synthesis in the intestine, but if the intestinal flora is suddenly changed (or destroyed by an antibiotic) the entire daily requirement must be supplied in the food.[32]

The second important protecting vitamin appears to be fat-soluble vitamin A. Experimental research has suggested that since hydro-carbons, viruses and radiations have all been shown capable of damaging the delicate enveloping membranes of certain enzymes within the cell, so that there is leakage of the enzyme material resulting in possible injury to some molecule with the survival of an abnormal cell, this damage to the membrane might be the crucial original stage in cancer production. It now appears that vitamin A protects against carcinogens at just this point by preventing damage to this highly important membrane. This discovery was reported to the International Cancer Congress in Tokyo in 1966 by Dr U. Saffiotti of the Chicago Medical School Institute for Medical Research giving strong support to the earlier suggestions that adequate vitamin A may enable cells to resist the effects of the powerful carcinogens producing lung, prostate and cervical cancer. Admittedly, this is still highly speculative, and the application to man of the experimental work carried out must be received with caution. Dr Saffiotti himself was extremely optimistic, and his further experimental work continues to show the same effects.[33,34] In view of our constant and universal exposure to the benzopyrenes (among the constituents of smoke held responsible for lung cancer) the prevalence in older men of prostate cancer, and the long waiting lists for cervical cancer, it would seem only sensible to examine closely our intake and absorption of vitamin A while awaiting fuller and further information.

There is a link here with the earlier stress on the importance of riboflavin and also of vitamin C*, for it has been known since 1939[35] that vitamin A can only be absorbed in the presence of adequate amounts of these two others. What matters, eventually, is not the intake, which may be inactivated or rejected by a body not

* Good sources are oranges, lemons, blackcurrants, tomatoes, sweet peppers, green leaf vegetables and sprouted seeds.

functioning properly for a number of reasons, but how much is actually absorbed in the intestine.

Sources of vitamin A
Animal foods such as dairy produce, liver, eggs and fish roe provide vitamin A as such, and vegetables such as green leaf vegetables, carrots, pumpkin and paw-paw provide it as the pro-vitamin carotene. On an average two to three times as much carotene as vitamin A is needed to give an equivalent value, but there are two qualifications for this statement: (*a*) only 1 per cent of carotene is absorbed from eating grated raw carrots, and cooking increases this up to 5–19 per cent. But juiced and drunk without delay to prevent destruction by oxygen, we get all the carotene as well as the catalase (see later paragraphs);[36] (*b*) since liver cells may not convert carotene to vitamin A as well as they should, it seems advisable to have other sources than vegetables, especially in illness.[37]

Some sources of vitamin or pro-vitamin A[38]

Excellent	Good	Fair	Poor	None
Fish liver oils	Watercress	Butter	Green peas	Sugar
Fish roe	Dried apricot	Egg	Cabbage	
Carrot	Spinach	Cheese	Herring	
Sweet potato		Green pepper	Banana	

Daily requirements of vitamin A and carotene mixed[39]

Man	Woman	In pregnancy	In lactation
5000 iu	5000 iu	6000 iu	8000 iu

Child	Boy	Girl
3000 iu	3000 iu	3000 iu

Daily requirements raised by: Pregnancy and lactation,[40] high fever and measles,[41] intake low in protein and high in refined starches, with impaired fat absorption through poor flow of bile,[42] exposure to long periods of strong artificial light or sunlight.[43] (Failure to see in a dim light may be a warning of a deficiency of this vitamin.)

N.B. Supplementation to excess by fish liver oils may cause toxicity, especially if there is an insufficiency of vitamin C.[44]

Robbers of vitamin A
The most prevalent thief is liquid paraffin, available without pre-

scription and very widely used as a laxative, in spite of strong evidence that it interferes seriously with the absorption of calcium and phosphorus as well as vitamin A and all the other fat soluble vitamins. It was strongly condemned in 1943 by the Council of the American Medical Association.[45] Also responsible for 'locking up' vitamin A are rancid fats, e.g. stale dripping, shelled nuts and stock pots, and oils not kept refrigerated after opening;[46] in the USA it appears that slightly rancid oils are often used in the preparation of cooking fats, margarine and vegetable oils which are not cold-pressed but extracted by a sort of dry-cleaning process;[47] reheated fats, much used in commercial and restaurant frying, which develop an anti-vitamin A factor;[48] low-fat diets followed in liver and gall bladder trouble and in slimming;[49] a deficiency of vitamin E (from a high extraction rate in white flour, or losses in cooking by roasting or frying at very high temperatures, and from an excess of lard in the diet);[50] iron compounds often taken in tonics and for anaemia[51] (though there are good natural sources in liver, kidney, apricots and green-leaf vegetables, which have no such drawback); aspirin found in almost every household and handbag;[52] pheno-barbitone frequently used as a sedative especially for migraine and epilepsy;[53] and cortisone given for arthritis and other conditions.[54]

It is of interest to note that breast milk contains from four to ten times as much vitamin A as cow's milk (there being of course a correlation with that present in the food eaten by the mother, bovine or human), underlining another great benefit of breast feeding.

Now for the factor of natural immunity. In his outstanding if partly controversial, *Soil, Grass and Cancer* (Crosby Lockwood, 1959), the late André Voisin stated that in his considered opinion, the one main objective of protective medicine must be to maintain the non-specific general immunity which has been called natural immunity. Seven years later an editorial review appeared in the *New Scientist* of the 43rd Annual Report of the British Empire Cancer Campaign for Research which contained information from nearly a hundred institutions and individuals to whom they have granted financial aid.

Surely a report from such a body must provide an excellent picture of the overall pattern of research in progress, ranging from molecular biology at one extreme to clinical trials of man-made drugs at the other. The review commented as follows:

'A noticeable feature is the growing interest in the immunological aspects of cancer. Not long ago reports of "spontaneous cures" have been regarded with scepticism, but many such occurrences have now been authenticated. There is increasing evidence that the body treats malignancies as "foreign" cells, reacting towards them just as it reacts towards bacteria, or a grafted kidney. Antibodies are produced, and other defence mechanisms are brought into play which tend to destroy the invader. It may be that we all develop cancers all the time, but that the abnormal cells evoke a response which brings about their own destruction, before they have had time to multiply and make their presence felt. *Frank, "clinical" cancers may only develop when the body's immune response is inadequate . . . If the central role of immunity is accepted, then it might be expected that people possessing a brisk defence mechanism would be the least likely to develop cancer.*'[55]

On what does this invaluable 'defence mechanism' then depend? Put as simply as possible it appears to rest on:

1 A healthy liver, capable of filtering out poisons and carcinogens. As a cancer expert has put it, 'Prevention of liver injury is identical with prevention of the disease [cancer].'[56]

2 A healthy reticulo-endothelial system consisting of cells in the spleen, lymph, liver and bone marrow, etc., which show a common behaviour in defence of the body through the phagocytes and leucocytes which attack any invader.

3 A healthy hormone system.

4 A protein (properdine) in the blood which, with its auxiliaries, fights against pathogens (disease producing materials), including carcinogens,[57] and magnesium plays a fundamental part in this.[58]

5 The conservation in our bodies of a high concentration of an enzyme (a substance corresponding roughly to the foreman who sees that work is carried out) christened 'catalase' in 1901.[59] This has been described as the 'fundamental defence enzyme' of living cells,[60] and is concerned with the catalase-peroxide balance of the body which is intimately connected with cancer.[61] How are we to keep these defence forces fighting fit to defend us?

Here is the opinion of the founder of the American Cancer Society: 'Since the major forms of cancer are largely the result of human habits and bad habits, *an intelligent reform of our habits* must be reached before cancer prevention can give tangible results.'[62] That is a general statement. Let us look at the details.

1 The liver quickly shows its disapproval of too much fat, as any

bilious sufferer knows. Emotional upsets, too, play a part, as we also learn if we give way to jealousy, anger or some other unfortunate emotion, making for extra bile. So, keeping on a steady keel and recalling the dictum of Sir Heneage Ogilvy about happiness, is our first task. Far more serious is the threat of the chlorinated hydrocarbons (DDT, PDCB, Dieldrin, etc.) which have the long-term effect of damaging the liver[63] and interfering with its normal ability to detoxify these and other harmful substances consumed in food and drink so universally today that there must be few with no impairment of liver functions.[64] Fortunately, however, a generous intake of vitamin C can protect the liver against highly toxic substances[65] without producing any of the unwanted side-effects of antibiotics.[66]

2 & 3 Both the reticulo-endothelial and the hormone systems depend for structure and maintenance on the materials with which they are supplied through what we eat and drink, so we must look to our nutrition.

4 In view of the widely prevalent programmes of heavy potassium fertilizing and of over-liming today (easily detected by such an observer as Dr Ehrenfried Pfeiffer on a visit to Britain) which unbalances the magnesium in the soil[67] unless it is given in the form of dolomitic limestone,[68] and the greatly reduced use of manures or compost, supplying the organic matter, without which magnesium may not be assimilable by growing crops,[69] many foodstuffs must be lacking this essential mineral today. Reliable sources are fruit and vegetables grown by organic methods; sea salt, with an analysis of chloride of magnesia 0·198 and sulphate of magnesium 0·067 parts by weight to 99·617 of sodium chloride and 0·118 sulphate of lime,[70] in place of refined common salt which contains no magnesium; and wholemeal compost grown flour at an extraction rate of 100 per cent which supplies 106 milligrams per 100 grams compared with a mere 13·9 milligrams in white flour at an extraction rate of 70 per cent.[71]

5 Unfortunately, catalase, present in nearly all plant and animal cells and therefore in food, is destroyed or inhibited by a very vast number of agents. These include chemical insecticides, fungicides, air pollutants, especially tobacco smoke, chemical additives to food and drink, sulpha drugs, barbiturates, certain tranquillizers and hormones, X-rays, cooking[72] and sodium fluoride now used for the compulsory fluoridation of water supplies, which a cancer expert has described as 'a potent catalase poison, and cumulative'.[73] Clearly,

yet another strong indication that all these factors are to be avoided
or curtailed.

Fortunately, however, there remain two simple ways of increasing
our own intake of catalase and its manufacture by our own cells.
The former by eating as many fruits and vegetables as possible, *raw*,
not cooked, as this destroys their catalase content. The latter by taking
plenty of daily exercise and exposing ourselves to that degree of
physiological stress which ensures that we react normally to such
normal stimulants as cold, obstacles and anxiety, so inducing by reflex
the synthesis of catalase.[74] Here individual amounts must be adjusted
to individual needs, for as someone has expressed it:

> *The thing for which we ought to press*
> *Is OPTIMUM amounts of stress,*
> *Though even dogs are hard to please*
> *With just the right amount of fleas.*

Sources of catalase in foods eaten raw [75]

Excellent	Good	Fair	None
Onion	Sweet pepper	Orange	Brewer's yeast
Banana	Tomato	Lemon	
Liver	Pear	Whole wheat	
Carrot	Apple	Cheese	
Egg yolk	Garlic		
Sweet potato	Maize		
	Melon		

Briefly summarized, the protective fence we can erect against the
onslaught of cancer consists of a healthy liver and a general defence
mechanism sustained by no smoking, great moderation in alcohol,
a minimum of refined sugars and starches, and hydrogenated (hardened) fats, and a watch on the weight, coupled with a daily diet
containing adequate amounts of riboflavin, vitamins A and C,
catalase and magnesium. As Dr Juan Zaffi with a lifetime of experience in the field of cancer patients has bluntly expressed it: 'It is
a question of choice. There are those who prefer cancer and their old
ways of preparing food, and those who prefer to spare themselves
cancer, accustoming themselves to a way of eating which can stave
off such a serious illness.' [76]

We are all free to choose fatalism for ourselves if we so wish but what right have we to choose fatalism for others? Do we or do we not care enough for the well-being of those who make up our households to expend the necessary effort to adapt our menus and our minds accordingly? Are we so content with the *status quo* that we intend to disregard the warnings of the experts, and wash our own hands of responsibility in this matter?

These are hard words to write as well as to read, but this is no subject for complacency—the issues are too serious. They demand some hard thinking and some yet harder, i.e. solid, action. Faced with the facts detailed earlier for our individual consideration, are we now prepared to act? It is surely more fruitful to act with faith and goodwill than do nothing with apathy.

Eric Linklater once wrote to the effect that if we are aware on the one hand of human suffering and on the other have some ability to lessen this suffering, we are 'doomed to action'. Let us not be doomed, but dedicated to action, to personal action to achieve such protection as lies in our power against cancer as could lead to its final prevention. As the Medical and Scientific Director of the American Cancer Society has pointed out, 'Only when everyone recognizes and accepts the importance of personal responsibility, will the control of cancer become a reality instead of the mere prospect it now is.'[77]

There can be no guarantee that the defences we have erected will not be breached, since cancer may not develop until many years after exposure to the carcinogen. According to the specialist, W. C. Hueper, some of the cancers observed at birth or in infants and children may be attributed to maternal exposure, while a cancer appearing in old age may have been caused in youth when small doses were encountered.[78] Nor can it be denied that taking the protective measures that have been enumerated entails taking thought, time and trouble, and means changing some cherished bad habits. None of us really likes doing this but even a disagreeable task seems a small price to pay for doing our best to protect our families from suffering which it may lie in our power to prevent. Then, should cancer come after all, we shall surely find the fortitude to face it for ourselves or for others with all that it entails, strengthened with the quiet assurance that we have not shirked our individual share in the common responsibility to cherish that well-being which fosters hope not fear. For as the Arab proverb tells us, 'He who has health has hope, and he who has hope has all.'

Tailpiece

The National Society for Cancer Relief, 47 Victoria Street, London SW1 issues a small publication *Not to Frighten but to Enlighten* which is sent free on application, and offers succour in the form of special nourishment, bedding, clothing, warmth or whatever may be required for any cancer sufferers unable to provide these things themselves.

REFERENCES

1   *Lancet* (6 July 1968)
2   MARTIN, W. C. *J. Appl. Nut.* (10 March 1957)
3   HUEPER, W. C. 'Environmental and Occupational Cancer', *Public Health Reports Suppl.* 209 (1948)
4   *Science* (16 June 1961)
5   BAUER, H. K. *Freiburger Symposium*, 249–60 (1954)
6   *New Scientist* (11 August 1966)
7   *Ibid.* (11 April 1968)
8   HUEPER, W. C. *J. Appl. Nut.*, 10, 149–165 (1957)
9   MAISIN, J. *et al. Rev. Belge des Sciences Medicales*, 13, 341–55 (1941)
10 BAUER, H. K. *Das Krebsproblem* (Berlin, 1949)
11 *Id., Freiburger Symposium*, 249–60 (1954)
12 VOISIN, ANDRÉ. *Soil, Grass and Cancer* (Crosby Lockwood, 1959)
13 KENSLER, C. J. *Cancer Research*, 7, 95–8 (1947)
14 MATTICE, M. R. *Bridges' Food and Beverage Analyses* (Henry Kimpton, 1950)
15 JOLIFFE, N. *New Eng. J. Med.*, 221–921 (1939)
16 HORDER, LORD, DODDS, C., and MORAN, T. *Bread* (Faber, 1954)
17 MATTICE, M. R. *Bridges' Food and Beverage Analyses* (Henry Kimpton, 1950)
18 *Manual of Nutrition* HMSO (1957)
19 WILLIAMS, R. J. *Am. Diet. Assoc.*, Vol. 36, 31 (1960)
20 JOLIFFE, N. *New Eng. J. Med.*, 221, 921 (1939)
21 KIMBLE, M. S. *et al. J. Biol. Chem.*, L11, 128, (1939) (Proc.)
22 MILLER, Z. *et al. J. Biol. Chem.*, 237, 968 (1962)
23 HORWITT, M. K. *et al. J. Nut.*, 39, 359 (1949)
24 DANIEL, ESTHER F. *Yearbook Separate No. 1681* of the US Dept. of Agric. (1940)
25 WILLIAMS, H. J. *et al. Science*, 96, 22 (1942)
26 SAPEIKA, N. *Actions and Uses of Drugs* (Balkema, Cape Town, 1955)
27 MICHELSON, O. *et al. Jour. Nut.*, 18, 517 (1937)
28 ELVEJHEM, C. A. *et al. JAMA*, 135, 279 (1947)
29 WILLIAMS, R. J. *J. Am. Diet. Assoc.*, Vol. 36, 31 (1960)
30 CALLOW, A. B. *Cooking and Nutritive Values* (Oxford University Press, 1945)
31 FREDERICKS, CARLTON, MD, and BAILEY, HERBERT, PHD. *Food Facts and Fallacies* (Julien Press, 1968)
32 ELVEJHEM, C. A. *Indust. and Engin. Chem.*, 33, 707 (1941)
33 SAFFIOTTI, U. *Cancer 20*, 857–64 (1967)
34 *Id. Am. Journ. Clin. Nut.*, Vol. 22, No. 8 (August 1969)
35 KIMBLE, M. S. *et al. J. Biol. Chem.*, 128, 52 (1939) (Proc.)

36 KREUTA, M. *et al. Nut. Abs. and Revs.*, X, 394 (1940)
37 *Nut. Rev.*, 7, 181 (June 1949)
38 MATTICE, M. R. *Bridges' Food and Beverage Analyses* (Henry Kimpton, 1950)
39 *Manual of Nutrition* (HMSO, 1955)
40 *Ibid.*
41 JOSEPHS, H. W. *Am. Jour. Dis. Child*, 65, 713 (1943)
42 WOHL, M. G., and GOODHART, H. S. *Modern Nutrition in Health and Disease* (Lea and Febiger, Phil,, 1965)
43 WISE, R. C. *et al. Ohio State Med. J.* 34, 666 (1938)
44 VEDDER, P. B. *et al. J. Nut.*, 16, 57 (1938)
45 AMERICAN MEDICAL ASSOCIATION COUNCIL. *JAMA*, 123, 967 (1943)
46 BURR, G. O. *et al. Phys. Rev.* 23, 256 (1947)
47 TOWNSEND, G. O. *et al.* Rancidity in Oils (Lee Foundation for Nutritional Research, Milwaukee, Wisconsin, 1943)
48 PEACOCK, P. R. *Brit. Med. Bull. 4*, 364 (1947)
49 HAND, D. B. *JAMA*, 181, 411 (1962)
50 MOORE, T. *Biochem. Jour.*, 34, 132 (1940)
51 REISMAN, K. R. *et al. Blood*, 10, 35–46 (1955)
52 SHAPIRO, S. *JAMA*, 125, 546 (1944)
53 DITCHBURN, R. W. *et al. Nature* 147, 445 (1941)
54 CLARK, I. *et al. Endocrinology*, 56, 232 (1955)
55 *New Scientist* (3 November 1966)
56 BLOND, KASPAR. *The Liver and Cancer* (John Wright, Bristol, 1960)
57 RHOADS, C. P. *et al. Proc. Am. Assoc. for Cancer Research*, 2, 251 (1957)
58 PILLEMER, L. A. *N.Y. Acad. of Science*, 66, 233–43 (1956)
59 LOEW, O. *US Dept. of Agric. Rept. No. 68* (1901)
60 VOISIN, ANDRÉ. *Soil, Grass and Cancer* (Crosby Lockwood, 1959)
61 HOLMAN, R. A. *Jour. Soil Assoc.*, Vol. II, No. 369 (1960)
62 CAMERON, CHARLES S. *The Truth about Cancer* (Hutchinson, 1957)
63 BISKIND, M. S. *Am. J. Dig. Dis.*, 20, 57–67 (March 1953)
64 JONES, R. J. *Nut. Rev.*, 21, 193 (1963)
65 WILLIS, G. C. *Can. Med. Ass. J.*, 76, 1944 (1957)
66 KLENNER, F. R. *J. Appl. Nut.*, VI, 274 (1953)
67 WALSH, T. *Potassium Symposium*, 327–52 (1954)
68 BEAR, F. E. *Soil Crop Science Soc. Florida* (17 October 1957)
69 *Id., Proc. Am. Soil Sci. Soc.*, 12, 380 (1958)
70 Maldon Salt Co. (Personal Communication)
71 HORDER, LORD., DODDS, C., and MORAN, T. *Bread* (Faber, 1954)
72 HOLMAN, R. A. *Jour. Soil Assoc.* (October 1960)
73 *Ibid.* (March 1962)
74 *Ibid.*
75 ZAFFI, JUAN. *Rev. Venez. de Sanidad y Asistencia Social*, XXVI, No. 1 (March 1961)
76 *Ibid.*
77 CAMERON, CHARLES S. *The Truth about Cancer* (Hutchinson, 1957)
78 HUEPER, W. C. *Southern Med. Jour.*, Vol. 50, No. 7, 923–33 (1957)

12

The Significance of Quality in Food

'Food is not merely an article of commerce and industry,
it is the stream of life itself.'

PROFESSOR SIR STANTON HICKS

Food not only plays a leading role as a defence against
cancer, it has been found that the quality of food affects the very
quality of life itself. The late Sir Robert McCarrison, formerly
Director of Nutrition Research, India, summarized the thesis of his
Cantor Lectures (1936) given before the Royal Society of Arts as
follows: 'The greatest single factor in the acquisition and maintenance
of good health is perfectly constituted food.'[1] It has been said of
this great pioneer of medical research nutrition that he began by
following the orthodox path of pathology, then turned instead to
study, not illness, but health, to try to discover its secret.

His conclusions were reached after a lifetime devoted to the study
of the effects of good nutrition compared with that of nutritional
deficiencies, and long years of feeding thousands of experimental
animals, mostly rats, on the actual national diets as prepared, cooked
and eaten by seven different races in India with whose physique and
capacities he was familiar.

The results show clearly that if the foods eaten supplied completely
all the elements necessary for normal nutrition, i.e. were perfectly
constituted, all the animals lived happily together, there were no
cases of illness, no maternal or infant mortality and no death from
natural causes over a period corresponding roughly to fifty years of
human life. On the other hand, those fed on the faulty foods of less
fortunate humans, such as the Madrassi of India or many in Britain
living on white bread, margarine, boiled potatoes and cabbage,
tinned meat and jam, with quantities of tea with little milk but much
white sugar, not only lived unhappily together, quarrelled and
became cannibalistic but mirrored all the diseases common to
humans similarly fed. In other words, faulty food upset the body's

function of nutrition, causing it to react in a number of unwanted ways, ranging from subnormal health to actual disease in many forms.

The right foods

Of what then does perfectly constituted food consist? According to Sir Robert, the essentials are whole grain cereals, milk and milk products (butter, cheese, sour milk, buttermilk, etc.), legumes (peas, beans, lentils, etc.), fresh root and leafy green vegetables with egg and meat occasionally, anything more being a matter of taste, and not of necessity. But there must be no omissions, and the amounts must be adequate, especially of milk and its products as well as of fresh vegetables, for these are the protective foods.

The requirements laid down by Sir Robert McCarrison have found general agreement in nutrition circles. In 1916 a United Kingdom government publication directed at the feeding of that key person, the munitions worker, stressed the importance of 'a sufficient quantity of nutritive material in proper proportions suitably mixed, easily digested, appetizing, attractive and obtainable at low cost'.

In 1959 the Council for Food and Nutrition of the American Medical Association summarized a balanced diet as follows:[2]

Group of foodstuffs	Daily requirements
Milk	Three to four cups for child and pregnant, two or more for adult.
Meat	Two or more servings of beef, veal, pork, mutton, fish, eggs, poultry, cheese, nuts, beans.
Vegetables and fruit	Four or more servings, including dark green or yellow vegetables, and citrus or other good sources of vitamin C fruit, as well as other vegetables and fruit.
Fats	Less solid fats than usual and mostly unsaturated, i.e. liquid oils.

The current *Handbook of Health Education* issued by the United Kingdom Department of Education and Science gave the same good nutritional advice.[3] Here are the precepts. Why are they so infrequently practised by those well able to afford them?

The chief reasons why so few today in an affluent society live on perfectly constituted foods appear to be the decline in soil fertility, with a lack of mineral balance in soils, the rise in food processing and fashions in food and the general ignorance of food values. Who are the healthy in the Western world today?

Certainly it is not the prosperous gentleman who booms 'Never had a day's illness' above the paunch of the stockbroker belt, with a coronary lying in wait after years of excess alcohol and high living largely on expense accounts; nor the anaemic woman who never stirs without her aspirins, peppermint tablets, laxatives and sleeping pills, though she may boast she never goes to the doctor. Still less is it the lollie-sucking and breakfastless child, with carious teeth and a built-in disinclination for exercise of muscle and mind. These are the uninformed unhealthy, but they and others can be restored to health with the wish for something better, the will to work for it, and the courage to be different from the unreflecting majority. Where to begin? Medical and agricultural experts tell us: in the soil itself.

Declining soil fertility
The dust-bowls and man-made deserts of the USA, Canada, Australia and Africa, the widespread destruction of the earth's surface owing to erosion and the decay of men and land where years of growing nothing but single crops have sucked the life blood of the soil, have become generally familiar, thanks to the many writers who have drawn attention to the doom they forecast. This general insidious fall in soil fertility, however seems to remain the concern of the few, although springing from the same causes—over-exploitation and a failure to return all plant and animal wastes to the soil from which they came—a simple conservation measure that was once almost universal.

Today, from drain, dustbins and stubble, we pollute our waters by discharging raw sewage into rivers and sea, and our air by burning wastes as we rob the soil of the humus it must have to produce nutritious foodstuff. As Sir Robert McCarrison has put it, 'The quality of foods themselves is important. This depends on the soil conditions in which they are grown, and on methods of cultivation, for if they are produced on impoverished soil the quality will be poor, and the health of those who eat them, man and his domestic animals, will suffer accordingly.'[4]

The over-enthusiastic use of artificial fertilizers has been shown by investigators to cause unbalanced protein formation, due to an over-forced diet causing plant indigestion and imbalance[5] although the advocates of such fertilizers have not failed to point out that 'the use of fertilizers in the absence of adequate supplies of humus is a misuse of fertilizers'.[6] Furthermore, a desire for quick returns and less labour (it is so easy to tip a chemical out of a sack), seems to have combined with Liebig's theory of mineral plant foods to *substitute* these chemicals for the age-old and proved practices of crop rotation, bare fallows and organic matter returned to the soil chiefly in the form of farmyard manure. Dr Ehrenfried Pfeiffer has pointed out that if the organic content of the soil drops below 1·7 per cent, leaching of minerals becomes very excessive.[7]

Unfortunately, the need of explosive manufacturers after the First World War to find other outlets for their factories equipped for the fixation of atmospheric nitrogen, gave an enormous impetus to this tendency to use chemicals rather than organic wastes. This was speeded up and intensified by the advertising described in general terms by George Santayana as 'the modern substitute for argument. Its function is to make the worse appear the better.' As a more recent observer has put it, 'The continued triumph of fertilizers has partly depended upon depreciating *quality* as an element in yield.'[8] (Author's italics.)

According to that eminent authority, the late Professor Dudley Stamp, 'The effect of artificial fertilizers, sprays, conditioners, etc., on the structure and the microfauna and microflora of the soil is unknown, and needs continuous study . . . Two lessons are outstanding, the ease with which delicate animal-plant balance is upset, and the complex chain reactions set up.'[9]

The importance of soil fertility for human health has been accepted by many of Sir Robert McCarrison's medical colleagues as is shown in the words of an editorial in the *Medical Press and Circular* of 1943: 'In this purse-proud capitalistic age, soil fertility is our one true capital, and soil health the one sure and lasting crop of public health in the widest and truest sense.'[10]

Quality soil builds quality food
Vigour or feebleness, health or disease begin in the bacteria of all soils, the roots of all plants and the mouths of all animals, and these three are inextricably interwoven in the cycle of nutrition. The bacteria need organic matter (humus), the plants need root-selected molecules, and the animals need matter which has been through either plants or other animals, in order to obtain the major and minor

minerals which are required in varying amounts by all living creatures. The living soil is the base of the pyramid of life, with plants
springing directly from it, animals growing indirectly from plants,
and man supreme at the apex, but yet dependent on the health of all
the rest for his own. Neglecting to copy nature and return all residues
to the earth to form humus to replenish it robs soil bacteria of their
rightful food, and deficient soils result, to be followed by deficient
plants and deficient animals, including man.

Man's responsibility for widespread soil deterioration is well
known. Less well known is the influence of shallow or deep roots on
the quality of the food provided by the plants they keep supplied with
nourishment, and the animals and men these in turn sustain. All
deep-rooted plants are able to bring up and incorporate in themselves minerals (and especially those called trace elements since they
are needed in only trace amounts) which may be largely inaccessible
to the shallow-rooted.

Tests have shown that meat from wild animals in East Africa
grazing on bush and woodland provides 23–29 per cent of poly-
unsaturated fatty acids as compared with the mere 2 per cent content
of domestic beef from Britain. The fat of wild buffaloes living in
woodlands in Uganda contained 30 per cent of unsaturated fats but
fell to 10 per cent if grazing was restricted to grassland.[11] Furthermore, the fat of domestic beef from Britain contained ten times as
much saturated fat as that of the wild buffalo, with three times as
much in the muscle meat.[12]

This confirms the finding of experts in the Second World War that
the best beef in Africa came from the Masai Reserve.[13] Not from the
shallow-rooted green grass pastures and confined pedigree cattle of
the European settlers, but from the native beasts of a primitive
pastoral tribe, cattle free to browse on a variety of deep-rooted
bushes, trees and weeds.

The Masai, themselves of outstandingly fine physique on their diet
of meat, milk and blood, supplemented with fruit and vegetables,
judge the value of a dairy cow by the time it takes her newly-dropped
calf to stand up and run; usually only a few minutes. This is deemed
necessary not only as a sure sign of vigour, but essential in the midst of
such predators as lions and hyenas. Calves from high-production
dairy cows in more sophisticated circles today are frequently unable
to stand for hours after birth, often for as much as twenty-four hours.
Their owners are only required to satisfy standards of butterfat

(saturated fat) with no standards for the vitally more important unsaturated fats, or the solids not fats (SNFs) indicating the minerals in the milk they sell.

If all British cattle were free to graze herbal leys (as used with so much success by the late Newman Turner, or today by Arthur Hollins and other organic farmers), and were to browse on bushes and weeds and trees in hedges and pastures, or were pastured on lucerne, as were the famous race-horses bred by the late Friend Sykes, and the Herefords and other breeds of cattle in Argentina, British beef could reach the highest standards of high mineral content coupled with low content of unwanted saturated fats. British dairy cows could also supply British children with the mineral-rich milk that builds fine bones and stamina rather than flabby fatties.

Much attention has been paid of late years to the composition and nature of fats in attempts to correct the abnormal fatty deposits known as atheroma in the walls of arteries, which are held to contribute largely to the occurrence of coronary attacks and other serious conditions.

The total protein content of modern meat has been increased by intensive rearing. Unfortunately, so has the saturated fat accompanying it. This is simply a source of energy and is not an essential food. Unsaturated fats, also called essential fatty acids (EFAs), on the other hand, are needed as building material for nervous tissue, blood and arterial visual walls which will accept no substitute. It has been demonstrated that the blood fats of people suffering from atherosclerosis consist mostly of saturated fats, while in those free from this disease they are mostly unsaturated fats.[14]

This throws light on the empirical preference of many housewives for eggs from free range or deep litter poultry rather than from battery hens. Although a recent report from the Cambridge School of Agriculture showed that eggs and embryos from free range poultry exhibited a greater variety of fatty acids and a larger amount of arachnidonic acid than those from batteries, this was dismissed as an 'academic distinction only', by the investigator.[15] Yet it had earlier been shown that the more arachnidonic acid in the blood of animals the more resistant they were to atherosclerosis, those species having a small proportion being liable to develop the disease spontaneously,[16] confirming a previous hypothesis that a deficiency of this fatty acid may be an important factor in the causation of atherosclerosis. Most of us would, therefore, be inclined to agree with the reviewer who pointed out that 'this finding seems sufficiently striking to indicate the need for further observation on the relevance to human disease, particularly atheroma'. Men have remade the hen, to the advantage of neither. They might be better occupied remaking themselves, by improving their own diet.

The wrong foods

It has been estimated that while two-thirds of the world is undernourished, the other third increasingly eats the wrong foods. Much of this can be attributed to the vast increase in food processing, for, as Dr F. A. Gilbert has pointed out, 'we can be protected by law against harmful drugs, but not against inferior and harmful foods'.[17] As far back as 1956 the impact of modern food technology on the nutrition of man and his domestic animals was expressed in the statement by experts that 'if it is accepted that processing includes all treatment of foodstuff from origin to consumption then barely 2 per cent of food [in calories] receives none'.[18] It should be emphasized that most processing consists either of subtracting valuable ingredients such as the germ of the wheat grain in order to sell it as an expensive supplement for stock or man, or in adding undesirable substances such as artificial colouring, flavours, etc., not enhancing nutritional quality, but in fact under suspicion as carcinogens. Both practices have been condemned by many medical and nutrition authorities, for instance by Dr E. J. Bogert in the words: 'Since refined foods such as highly milled grains have assumed a prominent place in the diet, ill-health due to vitamin deficiency has been frequent,'[19] and by the Rome Congress of cancer experts in 1956 (see Chapter 11) but they continue on their profitable course.

In addition, the growing popularity of television has brought with it the vogue of TV or convenience foods, thanks to the desire to spend as little time as possible away from the screen in preparing, cooking and serving meals. Unfortunately, these glamorously packaged, artificially coloured and flavoured substances bear little relation to Sir Robert McCarrison's perfectly constituted foods. Even today's potato crisps compare unfavourably with yesterday's chips. Once, a pennyworth of chips provided some cheap energy plus a little vitamin C; today threepence of the price goes to the upkeep of a modern factory whose product supplies not only negligible food value[20] but harmful substances owing to the high temperature of the frying fats which are used over and over again.[21]

Whole foods are quality foods
It now seems clear that what we eat should be governed not by chance or indifference but by conscious choice based on the ability to distinguish between non-foods, foods and whole foods. A consultant in Paediatrics has recently defined Wholefood as: 1 Balanced 2 Protective 3 Fresh 4 Wholesome.[22] This may be elaborated as follows:

1 *Balanced* and therefore compost grown, because artificial fertilizers used to excess to increase yields have been found to upset the amino-acid balance of the proteins[23] and in the case of wheat, the protein value is seriously limited by a low lysine content.[24]

2 *Protective* and therefore grown with organic matter, because growth-promoting factors including vitamin C were found by Sir Robert McCarrison in India in the 1920s and 1930s to be lower in plants grown with chemical fertilizers.[25] Later investigators reported that increasing nitrate fertilizers significantly reduced the vitamin C content.[26]

3 *Fresh* because wilting, storage and exposure to light after gathering reduce the content of riboflavin, pyridoxin and vitamin C.[27]

4 *Wholesome* (i.e. with nothing subtracted from or added to the natural product) because 'natural plant sources [of carbohydrate] contain both the fuel and the vitamin necessary for its complete breakdown to glucose [for energy], water and carbon dioxide'.[28]

The comfortable assumption that we in Europe are adequately supplied with this important vitamin B is unjustified. This was stressed by the late Sir Jack Drummond in a lecture given at the Royal Society of Arts just before the Second World War in these words: 'There is a firmly established view that the diets of Western Europe are sufficiently varied to include a sufficiency of vitamin B. I think this is a *very inaccurate and dangerous view to hold*. If one makes an analysis of a typical Western European urban diet, one finds that in every vital respect it is vitamin deficient and *probably in none more than* in vitamin B.' In the last forty years we have not improved this situation. Indeed, Dr Geoffrey Taylor has submitted striking evidence that today nutritional deficiencies which impair health, vitality and efficiency may be widespread at all ages. Clinical examinations carried out on numbers of children in schools, young men in the services and old people in hospitals and institutions have revealed a high percentage of cases showing the classic early symptoms of deficiencies of vitamins B_1 (thiamin), riboflavin, niacin, vitamin C and vitamin D.

Inadequate food and ill-treatment of food in the kitchen is held largely responsible, and it has been suggested that a clinical research unit with adequate biochemistry facilities should be set up by the Government to co-ordinate and carry out research into the relationship between low intake of vitamins and minerals, and health and disease.[29]

Such a common deficiency as that of vitamin B affects conduct as well as physical well-being as was stressed in 1957 at a symposium on nutrition at the School of Public Health at the University of Minnesota. It was stated in the published findings that a lack of vitamin B profoundly affects both the desire and capacity to work.[30]

A similar finding connecting food with mentality has since been revealed by the work of Dr John A. Churchill, Head of Research in child neurology at the La Fayette Clinic, Detroit, who, after studying twenty-two pairs of identical twins, stated that 'the placental circulation is not shared equally', each foetus does not get the same nourishment, and in each pair the heavier twin at birth had an IQ 5 per cent higher than the other. Rat experiments showed that on fat and protein deficient diets, as compared with a full diet, those litters on the former had a lack of development of the cerebral cortex [the grey matter of the brain] and were smaller at birth and duller. He drew the conclusion that 'not only the health but the mentality of the baby depends on eating a properly balanced combination of foodstuffs in pregnancy'.[31]

In these days, when we are surrounded by literally thousands of poisonous pesticides liberally used on farms, gardens and in homes with a National Poisons Information Service available for doctors, and forty-five hospitals in the British Isles able to provide them with emergency supplies of praxidoxine (P 2S) as a specific antidote in cases of poisoning due to organo-phosphorus compounds, it is interesting to recall the statement of an expert published in 1963 that 'the subject of nutrition has multifold significance for the clinical toxicologist. Good nutrition is protective against many poisons, notably hepatoxic [injurious to liver] substances. Whatever the causative agent, acute injury is accompanied by large losses of nutrients, while at the same time tissue damage creates extraordinary metabolic demands for many dietary factors'.[32] This confirms the opinion of the President of the American Medical Association expressed in 1959 that 'there is no better therapy today than a well balanced diet'.

Since there still appears to be some controversy whether wholefood is also health food, a small animal feeding experiment (SAFE) is currently under investigation as part of the Soil Association Haughley Experiment. Three groups of mice will be fed with grain from three experimental farms, which have been farmed consistently for more than twenty-five years to date. 1 with no artificial fertilizers but only self-produced compost. 2 with artificial fertilizers and farmyard manure and 3 with fertilizers only. A control diet of 'mouse nuts' will be fed to a fourth group. Some ten thousand mice per annum will be involved and detailed records will be kept of the long-term effects on the mice of these different methods of food cultivation.[33]

Men, however, remain more complex than mice. The best human food is that which frees us from preoccupation with physical ills to develop mental and spiritual capacities denied to the lesser animals. Unfortunately, whole foods may reach the eater heavily impaired by their passage through the kitchen.

This focuses attention on the important part played by the cook in the health of the nation.

REFERENCES

1 MCCARRISON, SIR ROBERT. *Nutrition and Health* (Faber, 1953)
2 WHITE, P. L. *Am. M. A. Council for Food and Nutrition* (May 1959)
3 *A Handbook of Health Education*. Dept. of Educ. and Science (HMSO)
4 SOIL ASSOCIATION film *'The Cycle of Life'*, Sir Robert McCarrison speaking
5 SCHUTTE, K. H. *et al. Nature*, 182, 958 (1958)
6 HOPKINS, DONALD. *Chemicals, Humus and the Soil* (Faber, 1945)
7 PFEIFFER, EHRENFRIED. *Soil Fertility, Renewal and Preservation* (Faber, 1947)
8 HULL, G. W. *Jour. of the Soil Assoc.* (April 1966)
9 STAMP, DUDLEY. *Council of the Brit. Assoc. for the Advancement of Science* (1960)
10 *The Medical Press & Circular 22*, Editorial. (12 September 1943)
11 *Lancet*, Editorial, 1, 1329 (22 June 1968)
12 *Ibid.*
13 KEONIG, OSKAR. *The Masai Story* (Michael Joseph, 1956)
14 LEWIS, B. *Lancet*, 2, 71 (1958)
15 JONES, D. *Nature*, 220, 921 (30 November 1968)
16 SWELL, L. *et al. Proc. Soc. Exp. Biol. & Med.*, 104, 325 (1960)
17 GILBERT, DR F. A. *Mineral Nutrition and the Balance of Life* (Univ. Oklahoma Press, 1957)
18 HOLLINGSWORTH, D. *et al. Proc. Nut. Soc.*, 15, No. 21, 2 (1956)
19 BOGERT, DR E. J. *Dietetics Simplified* (Saunders, 1954)
20 PYKE, MAGNUS. *Food Science & Technology* (John Murray, 1964)
21 BICKNELL, FRANKLIN. *Chemicals in Food and Farm Produce* (Faber, 1960)
22 WIGGLESWORTH, DR. McCarrison Soc. Meeting (London, 17 July 1966)

23 LAWRENCE, J. M. *Cereal Chemistry*, 35, 169 (1958)
24 MORANT, D. *Nut. Abst. and Revs.*, 29, 1–10 (1959)
25 MCCARRISON, R. *et al. Ind. Jour. of Med. Res.*, 19, 351 (October 1926)
26 KILGORE, L. *et al. Am. J. Clin. Nut.*, 14, 1 (1964)
27 MATTICE, MARJORIE. *Bridges' Food and Beverage Analyses* (Henry Kimpton, 1950)
28 *Ibid.*
29 TAYLOR, GEOFFREY. *Medical News* (30 July 1965)
30 REPORT *Am. Jour. Clin. Nut.*, 5 (1957)
31 CHURCHILL, JOHN, A. *Med. News* (4 March 1966)
32 GLEASON, M. N. *et al. Clinical Toxicity of Commercial Products* (Balton Williams and Wilkins, 1963)
33 *Observer* (8 December 1968)

13

Good Cooks and Good Health

'She who in these days of expensive living shows how the best use can be made of food material and who in any measure helps to revive what threatens to become a lost art in the home, does a work that far outweighs any within the power of woman.'

MARY HOOPER 1878

The selection, preparation, treatment and presentation of food before it reaches the eater vitally affects the destruction or preservation of its desirable qualities and this depends on the cook—the housewife in the kitchen. Indeed, if women were as food-conscious as they are fashion-conscious, possessing a good working knowledge of food values, rather than lack of interest, or even Cordon Bleu aspirations, we might well become a better fed, better tempered, better looking and healthier people. Cooking should not be regarded as a boring but necessary chore but as what it is, a highly responsible art, ideally to be carried on only by those aware of or ready to learn what really makes a good cook. On what should such a reputation be based? Patience, deftness, interest and the ability to follow a recipe with accuracy are obviously necessary, although the last attribute needs some qualification. Among the flood of would-be Beetons today (both Mr and Mrs) there seem to be very few who pay any attention to food values, and their luscious recipes in the Press too often add allure to harmful foods, to which we may be fatally attracted already. What child, or adult for that matter, needs pressing to eat pastries, sweet cakes, biscuits and desserts? It demands skill of course, to make such things, but is this skill used to the advantage of the eater? How much better for the cook to give up pandering to twisted taste buds and take up the challenge of *improving* them, so helping her household to relish and enjoy foods that are not only valuable nutritionally but can be made attractive by the knowledge and skill of a really good cook. Better to lavish time and trouble on an eye-catching salad than on curlicued cakes or meringues with lashings of cream.

The cook's choice
The first important decision made in the kitchen concerns the cook's choice of food and this must be based on a clear conception of what food is and why it is eaten.

Food is the source of proteins to build and repair the body cells, hormones to regulate its functions, enzymes, vitamins and minerals for digestion and maintenance, energy to be used in action, antibodies to protect against disease and genes to provide the next generation. Food is meant to make us glad, by promoting health, but too often it makes us sick and sorry, or even helps to kill us.

Good cooks know that some foods are better value than others; that highly refined and processed foods, though convenient because they keep, are dead foods that fail to support even a weevil or bacterium, much less a human being, and that it is foolish and may even be hazardous to provide only what an eater fancies or has been conditioned to fancy by skilful advertising.

There are loving wives who would feed their husbands on strychnine if they ate this with relish, and who go on swamping them with sugary health-stealers whose hidden robbery takes shape in irritability, overweight and worse as time goes on. Adelle Davis has confessed to being a poor hand at cakes. Coming from this Queen of Cooks, this confession underlines a popular fallacy. Cakes do not make cooks, nor good cakes a good cook. Cakes make fatties.

Indeed it takes little skill or intelligence to persuade the average person to eat or over-eat sweet and sugary foods. These are always attractive to infantile appetites, at whatever age. But foods prepared with the minimum of nutritional losses: succulent meats and fish; lightly cooked flavoursome vegetables, especially the green leaf kind; home-baked wholemeal bread and other delicious dishes not swamped with starch and sugar that are attractive to the eater yet keep him or her slim and healthy do testify to culinary capacity, and may be said to be the trade marks of a good cook.

To cook or not to cook
Perhaps the first decision to be made in every kitchen is what to cook and what to serve raw in a variety of inviting salads and desserts. With the exception of potatoes and quinces every single vegetable

and fruit can and should be eaten raw and a selection should be served at least once a day. At any rate a good portion of uncooked greenstuff should be eaten every day with hot or cold main dishes. Besides supplying optimum amounts of vitamin C, raw plants and cereals provide us with the catalase which is completely destroyed by cooking, yet is the enzyme important as offering us protection against cancer. (Chapter 11.)

In the Burma campaign of the Second World War soldiers were given the K diet, supplying in a dry form all the known constituents considered necessary but, if they were unable to obtain any raw food, they all developed sprue in a few days.

However, there are foods which must be adequately cooked for safety. These include beef, pork, fish and egg white. Imperfectly cooked beef may contain the larval form of the common tapeworm (*Taenia saginata*), which develops into the adult in the intestine of the eater.[1] Adequately cooked pork or sausage meat should look grey and have lost all trace of redness. If not properly cooked, and coming from a pig suffering from the round worm *Trichinella spiralis*, it can cause outbreaks of trichinosis, resulting in muscular pains and other unpleasant symptoms as the embryos pass into the tissues, and these may continue for several weeks until the larvae in the muscles finally calcify.[2]

Infection by the fish tapeworm *Diphyllobothrium latum* occurs from raw or imperfectly cooked fish and can cause pernicious anaemia since the parasites are avid for vitamin B_{12}. Among fish harbouring the infective stage are salmon, pike, perch and trout.[3] The thiaminase present in herring, carp, clams, lobster, mussels, shrimps and cockles, if eaten raw, destroys thiamin (vitamin B_1) in the eater.[4] Smoked fish are also listed among possible carcinogens in *The Prevention of Cancer* by R. W. Raven and Francis J. C. Roe (Butterworth, 1967).

Raw egg white is known to inactivate biotin, one of the vitamin B complex, but need not be wasted when using the yolk to make mayonnaise. It can be added to any form of cooked egg, except, of course, a boiled one.

What cooking will not do
Cooking makes animal foods palatable, but there are some things it cannot do. Among these are the following: cooking cannot

1 Destroy nitrates present in foods from farm effluents or chemical fertilizers which change to nitrites in the body.[5] Since these can be

dangerous for babies, it is best to avoid all commercial strained baby vegetables and steam then sieve compost grown vegetables for any infant.[6]

2 Remove or neutralize residues of persistent pesticides.

3 Destroy any noxious additives such as the dyes in processed peas. This is what Dr Werner Schuphan, Director of Federal Research Institute of Plant Products, Geisenheim, Rhine, has to say on the subject: 'Even at the present time one finds "poisongreen" coloured canned peas in the British Isles, and to these the British consumer does not appear to object.'[7] Incidentally, these are the peas almost invariably served in restaurants as their one green vegetable.

It is important to remember when preparing any vegetable for use raw that airborne dust may contain particles of the excreta of dogs, cats or farm animals, bringing a risk of salmonella infection, which gives rise to the so-called 'food-poisoning' that affects thousands every year in Britain. This may also be due to under-cooked meat or stale sausages, or pies and cakes filled with cream.

Getting the best value from fruit and vegetables
The rules for preparing vegetables and fruit are simple and few, but important. It is so easy to be a killer in the kitchen, murdering the enzymes, vitamin and minerals committed to our care and necessary for the health of the household. Here is a list of the essential rules and the reasons for them.

Rule	*Reason*
1 Leave on roots, tops and outer leaves in gathering or buying. Cut off just before washing.	Delays wilting, and vitamin values are increased until the onset of wilting, when they decline.
2 Wash rapidly and thoroughly under the cold tap.	Soaking or using warm water causes loss of vitamins B and C.
3 Drain quickly, then pat fruits and roots dry with Turkish towelling. Dry leafy ones by whirling in a bag made of this or an old pillow slip.	This prevents minerals, water soluble B and C and flavours passing into the water as readily as sugar or salt.
4 Keep in a plastic bag, or other closed receptacle in refrigerator until required for salads or cooking.	Prevents attack by oxygen and enzymes causing loss of vitamins A, C and E.

Rule	Reason
5 Keep all requiring storage in a cool dark place.	Light and warmth can steal much riboflavin, folic acid and vitamin C.
6 Avoid peeling as much as possible.	Many valuable nutrients lie in and under the skin.
7 Never discard liquids from cooking. Save for use in soups and gravies.	These contain extracted minerals and vitamins.

A salad for all seasons

Anglo-Saxon husbands often include he-men who scoff at raw green leaves as mere 'rabbit-food'. Their Continental brothers, choosing to eat a daily salad with any dish, hot or cold, need no telling that even a superficial look at the private life of the rabbit reveals an outstanding virility.

According to *Chambers Twentieth-Century Dictionary*, a salad is 'a preparation of raw herbs (lettuce, endive, chicory, celery, mustard and cress, water cress, onion, radishes, tomatoes, chervil, etc.) cut up and seasoned with salt, vinegar, etc.', showing that although cold potato and Russian salads are useful ways of using left-overs, they are not entitled to call themselves salads.

We can expand this list of raw herbs so as to provide a real salad daily throughout the year without paying exorbitant prices for any out-of-season ingredients. It is monotonous to use lettuce as the only green leaf and can be ruinously expensive in winter, and there are not only many other green leaves which offer far better value, but many roots and fruit vegetables which can supplement them or take their place.

Pigs going short of vitamin C because their food contains none or has been over-cooked show this by losing the curl in their tails. A pity perms do not react in the same way. What a health-and-beauty-building run that would cause on salads, which are excellent sources of carotene, vitamin C and folic acid, as well as catalase and lysine, both essential nutrients destroyed by cooking.

Spring. Available for salads

Leaves Mustard, cress, summer spinach, lettuce, chives, parsley, mint, lemon balm, garlic mustard (*Alliaria petiolata*), watercress, chick-weed (*Stellaric media*), dandelion (*Taraxacum officinale*)

Flowers or fruit   Broccoli, cauliflower, sweet peppers
Roots   Spring onions, radishes

Summer. Available for salads
Leaves   Lettuce, cabbage (Summer Monarch cabbages—the nicest raw), parsley, mint, lemon balm, watercress, chives, savoy, nasturtium
   Flowers or fruit   Cauliflower, broccoli, ridge cucumber, young peas, tomatoes
   Roots   Beet, leek, radish, carrot

Autumn. Available for salads
Leaves   Cabbage (Autumn Monarch), celery, savoy, endive, lettuce, dandelion, red cabbage
   Flower or fruit   Tomatoes, broccoli
   Roots   Beet, carrot, kohlrabi, parsnip, radish, turnip, swede

Winter. Available for salads
Leaves   Cabbage (Winter Monarch), red cabbage, endive, dandelion
   Flower or fruit   Broccoli
   Roots   Carrot, beet, turnip, swede, parsnip

How to use leaves
Pick freshly, wash rapidly but thoroughly, dry in salad basket or clean dry cloth gathered up by the four corners and swished about until all the moisture has gone. Tear soft leaves, and shred hard ones with sharp knife, put in deep bowl and incorporate chosen dressing until leaves are coated. Serve at once with wooden servers or spoons.

If gathered on warm day, put in refrigerator for an hour or so in closed plastic bag before preparing. Chives, parsley, mint or lemon balm cut into small pieces with kitchen scissors can be sprinkled over or served in separate bowl to be added according to individual taste.

Perhaps the most useful spring leaves are the thinnings from a row of summer spinach, which braves the weather holding the lettuce back. Eaten very young, about two inches long, these are sweet and delicious, for, judging by the flavour, it seems the oxalic acid has not yet risen in them.

How to use flowers or fruit
Broccoli and cauliflower need careful washing and drying. Sprigs

can then be broken into easy-to-handle bits and served with small bowls of mayonnaise for dipping, or treated as leaves and coated with the desired dressing in a large bowl. Incidentally, cooked cauliflower has a higher vitamin value than the raw material.

If ridge cucumbers are well-washed they can be sliced with the peel still on and this prevents them from being indigestible. Sousing them with vinegar spoils the delicate flavour so it is better to add some oil and sprinkle with mint or parsley. Green peas in their youth should never be cooked, but make a delicious addition to any salad. Sweet peppers must have their very pungent seeds removed before use, and must not be confused with the hot variety used in pickling. Those who find them indigestible should eat them in moderation.

Roots

Roots stored in dry peat are invaluable for winter salads. Beet, turnip, swede and carrot can all be taken up, dried off and brushed clean of soil, then stowed between layers of dry peat in a tea chest, standing on jampots if rats are a possibility, as they cannot climb up the glass. Raw shredded carrots are commonplace, but contain less food value than cooked carrots, though pleasant and popular. Raw shredded beets are better because they contain betaine which can double for choline (part of vitamin B complex) which is likely to be short if too little protein is eaten, and is needed to help the body utilize fat. Cooked for ages and drowned in vinegar they lose half their charm. Scrub and if necessary peel, then shred or grate. Kohlrabi, onions, leeks—using about three inches of the green part—and spring onions, can all be sliced and served in separate bowls, since they are not to everyone's taste. Soaking all the onion family in oil and refrigerating for half an hour or so removes the 'repeater' action.

Wild salads

The advantage of these is that they cost nothing and can be found when there is nothing yet available in the garden or prices are high in the shops. Well-washed chick-weed, choosing leaves which are large and tender before flowering begins, and placed between slices of home-made bread and Marmite makes sandwiches which children like as well as adults. As one of its other names reveals, 'Jack in the hedge' (*Alliaria petiolata*) or garlic mustard, is to be found in many hedges in spring and adds a pleasant garlicky touch, much milder than the clove garlic. Most French markets sell dandelion leaves for salad, but we in Britain have to look for our own *Taraxacum offici-nale*, though they are usually not far off. Choose young leaves, for they get bitter in their old age.

Salad dressings
Liquidized mayonnaise: 1 raw egg yolk; 1 teaspoon honey; 1 table-spoon lemon juice; pinch of salt; up to 8 ozs oil (sunflower, corn or peanut are more valuable than olive). Put the egg, honey and vinegar in the liquidizer and turn to lowest speed, with baffle and lid on, but omitting centre covering. As it spins slowly pour oil through this hole. Stop adding oil when it has thickened to your taste. This can be stored in the refrigerator for a few days in a screw-topped bottle. Mustard and pepper can be added to taste.

Cheaper version: 1 dessertspoon boiled potato; 1 tablespoon cream or top of the milk; 1 saltspoon salt; 1 teaspoon brown sugar; 1 dessertspoon lemon juice. Mix the potato, sugar and salt smoothly and add cream gradually. When smooth stir in lemon juice drop by drop.

Cooking vegetables
Boiling vegetables is an insult to plant and palate and should never be inflicted on either. Methods of preserving flavour, appearance and food value include the following:

1 Absolutely accurate pressure cooking according to the instruc-tions issued with the utensil. Over-cooking very rapidly occurs causing unpleasant odours leading to flatulence and indigestion from the breakdown of sulphur, destruction of vitamin B complex as well as vitamin C, and loss of flavour through expulsion of aromatic oils and damage to proteins.

2 So-called waterless cooking. This in fact requires a couple of tablespoons of water heating to boiling point to fill the utensil with steam to drive out the oxygen. When the material is heated through, heat is lowered to prevent escape of steam and the natural water con-tent is sufficient to complete the cooking.

3 Steaming in a steamer or on a rack in a pan. Vegetables are left unpeeled and uncut if possible to prevent too many minerals and water soluble vitamins dissolving into the water below, which should in any case be kept and used in gravy or soup.

4 Sautéing in a covered pan. Heat 1–2 tablespoons of oil. Well dried and chilled vegetables are shredded freshly with a sharp, stain-

less steel knife, dropped in and well tossed to coat them with the oil, and seal the surfaces against oxygen. When heated through, they should cook at lower heat about five to ten minutes in their own juice.

5 Grilling after brushing with oil, heating rapidly to heat through, then turning low to ensure crispness and to prevent shrivelling.

6 Baking either in or out of jacket for onions as well as potatoes, beetroot and parsnips. This has the disadvantage of slow initial heating and long cooking, with subsequent loss of vitamin C and more still if jacket is removed by peeling and exposure to oxygen. This can be overcome to some extent if surfaces are brushed with oil, or if first steamed and only finished in pre-heated oven.

7 Short cooking in milk. Milk, like oil, acts to prevent dissolution of minerals, etc., and has a wonderfully sweetening effect on even quite elderly leaves of cabbage, red and white, cauliflower, broccoli, chard, kale, spinach (any variety), tops of turnips and radishes, etc., and also such sulphur-rich things as onions, turnips, and cauliflower curd that often cause digestive distress. This is the method, advocated by Adelle Davis. It is wise to brush the bottom of the pan with oil to prevent the milk catching, which it does so easily if one turns one's back. After applying the oil, pour in $\frac{1}{2}$–1 cup of milk, replace lid and bring to steaming point. Meanwhile shred the vegetable with a sharp knife or cut up small if a root, drop it in, replace lid, shake well to coat all surfaces with the milk, keep heat up for a few seconds to heat through, then lower to simmering and leave 5–7 minutes. If all the milk has not been absorbed, pour it off to add to gravy or soup, and serve the vegetable as it is.

N.B. To prevent over-salting, sprinkle with a pinch of sea salt just before serving and garnish with paprika, chopped fresh herbs, a dash of oil or butter, or a grating of onion, as liked.

Meat cookery

Meat-lovers usually need little pressing to eat meat in spite of any nutritional errors committed in the cooking. These can and should be avoided. High temperatures always toughen proteins, and in pressure cooking may do them damage, and over-heated fats used in frying and over-roasted and over-grilled meats can be carcinogenic.[8] Therefore, all meats are best cooked slowly at low temperatures. Such cooking produces tenderness, less shrinkage and more succulence which increase the flavour. For a pleasantly browned surface without over-cooking, wholemeal flour or crumbs, paprika, molasses or non-instant powdered milk may be used, and basting with vegetable oil which serves to keep in the juices.

Less expensive than joints and steaks are cheaper cuts of less tender meats; elderly rabbits, stewing fowls, and so on, braised or casseroled at low temperatures for long periods, to retain flavour and produce the desired tenderness. Better value nutritionally are the internal organs headed by liver and including heart, kidney, sweetbreads and brain, which can all be served in a variety of inviting ways. Because poultry contains less fat and is more quickly digested, it is often prescribed in illness but is of no higher food value than any other flesh food.

Those eschewing flesh foods need more than the average knowledge of nutrition to obtain a balanced diet. Merely cutting out all meat, fish, eggs and dairy products is not vegetarianism, and may lead to disaster if only unselected plant foods are eaten. Soya beans, peas, lentils and peanuts, in fact, contain more protein than an equal weight of milk, or meat, but need supplementation by leaves and seeds to make them complete proteins. Nuts are the best meat substitute in a concentrated form. Coconut, however, has little food value compared with walnuts, almonds, brazils and others. These are all expensive, and can be indigestible unless lightly browned and milled or grated.

Fish cookery
So far fish remains more wholesome than meat, since it is untouched by man-administered hormones or antibiotics, although pesticides have reached it through the plankton on which it feeds. Roman Catholics who eat fish on Fridays from religious principles may regard this as a penance, but it is good nutritional practice. In common with all seafoods it supplies the iodine essential for the thyroid gland, with an increased need in pregnancy and lactation, when it is passed on to the growing child. After the First World War, when fish was not only scarce but expensive, there were many women with enlarged thyroids. There is less iodine in freshwater fish, but salt-water fish eaten two or three times a week should provide sufficient, and vegetarians should use iodized table salt or seaweed products.

Fish contains about the same amount of protein as meat, with a comparable content of the essential amino-acids, and being active creatures they are rich sources of vitamin B complex. However, this is easily lost if the skin is stripped off and the fish is cut, washed slowly and left wet or cooked in any fluid which is discarded. Fish preserved in brine, which must be soaked out overnight, cannot be commended nutritionally either.

The cooking of fish differs from meat cookery in that it depends not on poundage but on thickness. As soon as the internal temperature reaches 140°F the raw flavour is lost as the proteins begin to get firm, and they continue to get firmer as the heat increases. To ensure against over-cooking and also to prevent unpleasant odours in the house, this temperature should not exceed 150°F.

The common practice of boiling fish is not only guaranteed to prejudice anybody against fish for ever, but soaks out all flavour and most of the food value, and it is difficult to steam or stew without over-cooking, which leaves it dry and flavourless. The most rewarding ways are baking, grilling, casseroling and creaming. When baking fish, it is best to place it on a wire rack in a baking dish so that it is surrounded by dry heat. Grilling can be used for any fish not more than an inch thick, and creaming by adding diced raw fish to a sauce or casserole that is hot but not quite boiling three minutes before serving. This keeps the flavour and runs no risk of over-cooking.

A better method than frying is to sauté fillets or steaks of fish in a hot pan brushed with oil and left uncovered. Nutritionally, deep fat frying is not to be commended. The fish is usually dried out, the calories supplied are excessive, and the fat is overheated, causing destruction of vitamin E, and damaging the vitamin B complex and vitamin A content of the fish. Furthermore, the solid saturated fats generally used may elevate the blood cholesterol, and using the fat again and again may develop an anti-vitamin factor which destroys part of the vitamin A activity of foods eaten at the same time.[9] Vegetables such as tomatoes, onions, carrots, etc., quickly cooked, combined with a sauce prepared in the same utensil and raw fillets or diced fish added make delicious casseroles cooked in a slow oven (325°F about 12 minutes).

Hang on to breakfast
We should all have Barrie's words 'Hang on to breakfast' framed on our kitchen walls as a reminder to discourage breakfast skippers and tea and toast bolters. Studies have been made on the subject at many universities and tests have shown the value of eating one quarter to one third of the day's food at the first meal of the day when muscle efficiency is at its lowest.[10] Old and young, fat and thin thrive best on an adequate breakfast which establishes the blood sugar level

determining our energy and how we think, act and feel. If breakfast is high in protein, and low in fat and starch, digestion is slow and energy is maintained at a high level for many hours to follow.[11] This is especially important for children.

The firmest basis for what Isaak Walton called a 'good honest hungry breakfast' is a good appetite. Adults who cannot eat anything in the early morning are tacitly confessing to having overindulged in food, alcohol or tobacco at the last meal of the previous day, which should have been a light one. It is a pity a child's naturally hearty appetite should be fobbed off with a dash of milk, a smother of white sugar and a plateful of the highly processed contents of some carton. This supplies a minimum of protein, and an excess of carbohydrate sending the blood sugar racing up, to fall again rapidly, causing a feeling of fatigue and a craving for sweets, long before the next meal is due.

An egg quickly cooked in a variety of ways, a chunk of cheese, liver or bacon, or yeast extract with wholemeal bread and butter and a glass of milk provide good protein fat and carbohydrate, taking little time to prepare and no longer to eat than the over-sweet cereal and give the longest lasting energy. A smaller helping of cereal (with milk and a dash of honey) might be permitted after the good protein has been eaten but this is far better omitted and an apple or raw carrot would be a better addition.

Wholemeal is basic
For vegetarians, as for all those wishing to eat not only the best but the most deliciously flavoured bread and flour products, wholemeal is basic for all purposes where flour is employed. The emphasis on whole does *not* mean eating the husks like a modern prodigal son. It means that only the inedible husk is discarded, leaving the grain with all its ingredients intact. During milling and refining to make white flour over twenty substances including the most valuable proteins, vitamin E, the vitamin B complex and many minerals are removed, and a fraction of three of these substances put back as a so-called 'enrichment'. No wonder using wholemeal breadstuffs pays nutritional dividends. Such wholemeal bread can be bought, but it is easily out-classed by a good home-made bread.*

* A booklet entitled *Basic Food Guide* which includes an easy recipe for wholemeal bread is obtainable free from Henry Doubleday Research Association, Bocking, Braintree, Essex, on receipt of a s.a.e.

'The defects of a white bread, white sugar, meat and potato type of diet can be made good by two types of protective foods—milk and green leafy vegetables' according to a well-known nutrition expert, Professor E. V. McCollum. Anyone forced by institutional living, an uncooperative family, or other circumstances, to eat such defective foods, can offset their disadvantages by providing themselves with extra milk and yogurt and cress, water cress, or other green leaves to be eaten raw. Furthermore, adding small amounts of powdered debittered brewer's yeast—selected by the US Navy as the food out of the hundreds available to be stored in all lifeboats and rafts—to such foods as gravies, enables some of the large surplus of vitaminless starches and sugars to be broken down in the body to glucose for energy, with carbon dioxide and water to be excreted as waste.

By choosing food well and conserving all its nutritional values by careful treatment and cooking, a good cook not only plays a vital part in the conservation of food resources which form an intimate part of everyone's environment, but contributes largely to the wellbeing and health of a household, and so of a nation.

REFERENCES

1 BLACKWELL, D. B., and SOUTHWELL, T. Guide to Parasitology (H. K. Lewis, 1961)
2 RANSOM, B. H. et al. Jour. Agri. Res., 17, 201–21 (1919)
3 SCHRIMSHAW, N. S. et al. WHO Monograph, 57 (1968)
4 DESROSIER, N. W. The Technology of Food Preservation (AVI Pub. Co. Inc., 1963)
5 KILGORE, L. et al. J. Am. Diet. Assn., 43, 39 (1963)
6 WILSON, J. W. Agron. Jour., 41, 20 (1949)
7 SCHUPHAN, DR WERNER. Nutritional Values in Crops and Plants (Faber & Faber, 1961)
8 RAVEN, R. W., OBE, TD, FRCS, and ROE, FRANCIS, J. C., DM, DSC PATH, MC., The Prevention of Cancer. (Butterworth, 1967)
9 PEACOCK, P. R. Brit. Med. Bull, 4, 364 (1947)
10 ORENT-KEILES, E. et al. US Dept. of Agri. Circular No. 827 (1949)
11 THORN, G. W. et al. Anns. Int. Med., XVIII, 913 (1943)

14

The Need to 'have a Concern'

'The most important possession of a country is its population. If this is maintained in health and vigour, everything else will follow. If this is allowed to decline nothing, not even great riches, can save the country from eventual ruin.'

SIR ALBERT HOWARD

There are those who will question the emphasis in the preceding chapters on the prevention of ill-health and the achievement of good health as an eminently desirable goal. The most succinct reply to this criticism comes in the words of Emerson: 'Give me health and a day and I will make the pomp of Emperors ridiculous', health being taken to consist of physical, mental and moral strength and balance.

Confirmation of this earlier opinion was expressed by the Soil Conservation Department of FAO at Washington in 1968: 'Good health increases ambition and confidence in the future, which can only lead to an intensified concern for an unsullied maintenance of resources.' No need, today, to stress the importance of a readiness to be concerned over conservation and pollution.

For a long time medical men themselves have been dissatisfied with the failure of their profession to concentrate on the prevention rather than on the treatment of disease. This attitude was clearly summed up by Dr H. Beric Wright, in his book *Fit for Life* (Evans, 1968), 'Britain has a National Health Service, but heaven knows how it got its name for none of it is preventive, and all its agencies— general and special hospitals and family doctors—spend their whole lives treating illness and disease.'

It was encouraging that delegates to the 23rd World Health Assembly held in Geneva in May 1970 condemned the traditional methods of training doctors at universities and teaching hospitals, pointing out that although a high percentage of patients suffered from preventable disease, there was no emphasis in the curriculum on prevention, to which insufficient attention was paid. Were this to be remedied, the general fatalistic approach to ill-health might gradually disappear as we all learn that good health largely depends on our own conditions and habits.

Contesting all the dangers that may assail us in daily life stands our vital force, our inner core, a living instrument that can defy them all. If this is strong we can face any foe, though we need all its powers to use our abilities and latent capacities to the full. Why be content to dissipate them in unnecessary struggles with remediable dangers in our immediate personal environment? Why not remove or reduce these dangers? Previous chapters have suggested how this could be done, although not without taking thought. Above all, we must beware of complacency. This inevitably breeds catastrophe, and eternal vigilance remains the price of safety.

It is the duty of the State to ensure public safety. In our personal lives we must accept that this duty falls on us, and that home is the domain where health and freedom from preventable perils is the concern of the home-maker and the head of the family. Concern for a wider environment comes next, and here we can and should lend a hand.

An invocation intended to be added to the Church litany, once hopefully drawn up by the Council for the Preservation of Rural England, contained this plea: 'From all polluters of earth, air and water . . . from all foul smells, noises, and sights, good Lord deliver us!' It is surely as worthwhile an aim to preserve and remake the national health in mind, body and estate, as to preserve rural England as part of a general conservation and anti-pollution programme.

Projects in European Conservation Year
It has been claimed that in 1970 Britain took the lead in 'world-wide stirring of man's conscience to fight the disease of pollution'. Some two thousand projects were planned to give people a wider understanding of the problems, with conferences, lectures and films being given up and down the country.

In May, the British Government itself published a White Paper called *The Protection of the Environment—the fight against pollution* (HMSO). Owing, however, to the timing of the General Election, this proved to be a premature delivery which disappointed many who had expected a full-scale survey and had to be satisfied with an undersized document.

Suggestions for what organizations and individuals could do to improve Britain's environment were well set out by a free booklet called *European Conservation Year. United Kingdom. 1970.* (Available from the Nature Conservancy, 19 Belgrave Square, London SW1.)

In America, students had already turned their attention to environmental pollution. In 1969, Texas University formed a Legal Organ for the Protection of the Environment (nicknamed the 'Chlorophyll Conspiracy'), and Columbia an Ecology Action Group. So perhaps 1970 will indeed go down in history as 'the year mankind stopped letting things happen', in the hopeful words of Prince Philip.

In 1969 comprehensive plans for saving the planet were detailed in a book by Max Nicholson, Director of the Conservation Section of the International Biological Programme. This was described by John Davy, in a review, as a kind of handbook for the new age, a first primer for the formidable educational task of overcoming the ecological illiteracy which still abounds in industries and governments all over the world. Obviously this task will take time. We must not wait for the authorities to act. We must act ourselves, even if with but modest results. Where is the money to come from? Professor Goran Lofroth of Stockholm University has provided the answer in plain blunt terms, 'The cost of protecting the environment ought to be paid before we are allowed the luxury of consuming relatively unnecessary goods.'

Yet there are still many who will object that reform will cost too much, that freedom from pollution is something only the wealthier nations can afford, instead of an inalienable human right. The Council of Europe at the European Conservation Conference, held at Strasbourg in February 1970, thought otherwise and said as much quite plainly. A Declaration was issued proposing that the Council of Europe be charged to draw up a protocol to the European Convention on Human Rights guaranteeing the right of every individual to enjoy a healthy and unspoiled environment—this protocol to cover the right to breathe air and drink water reasonably free from pollution, the right to freedom from undue noise, and other nuisances, and to reasonable access to coast and countryside. Furthermore, it was stated that the major environmental issues in Europe and other highly industrialized regions were:

1 Planning of the natural environment and its resources.
2 Elimination, disposal and re-use of modern society's by-products and wastes, recycling of by-products and wastes to be given special attention.
3 The use of poisonous substances.

The conclusion reached was that *'these issues can only be resolved if individuals, aware of what is at stake, feel personal responsibility for their environment'*. (Author's italics.)

Here the Council has really got down to grass roots and given us all a clear directive.

Rules, regulations and penalties can force us to restore to health the vast areas of earth, air and water we have irresponsibly polluted, and to aim at the conservation of resources we have plundered in the past. They can *not* force us to restore to health our own diseased sense of values—perhaps the most prevalent form of ill-health in modern times—so that we recover a sense of personal responsiblity to carry out the necessary rehabilitation. It is our sense of values that makes us men, not merely primates. Lacking a true sense of values, we become blind to the basic need to protect our heritage of life. Science has given us the knowledge to see our mistakes with their grave consequences. Science has told us what we can do to remedy them. Only a new standard of priorities can convince us that we *ought* to remedy them, and without loss of time. Increasingly and almost imperceptibly we have poisoned and polluted our world, and present generations are paying the price. This need not and must not be the legacy we leave behind. Perhaps the most difficult problem in this situation is how best to develop and maintain human beings who are whole and healthy in spirit and therefore ready to practise control and responsibility over themselves, and over-all they hold, or should hold, in trust for future generations. How are we to impress on ourselves and on others, our human obligation, as temporary stewards, not owners, of all earth's resources in land, sea, air and water, to hand down not a worse but a better world to those who succeed us?

Man before Moon
France has sent no man to the Moon. Instead, with traditional commonsense and an admirable sense of immediacy, she has chosen to work on presenting the world with the first blueprint for a pol-lution-free city. The site selected is Vaudreuil near Rouen, and the

project is under the direction of M. Jean Ternisien, a physicist and metallurgist with considerable industrial experience. Becoming impatient with the remedial approach to pollution problems, he argued that to start from scratch would teach scientists much more than dealing with existing urban agglomerations. With fifty-seven specialists reporting to him, M. Ternisien is working out the ground rules. The terms of reference cover everything from atmospheric conditions to the existing laws relating to environmental interference, and the final report is to be distributed to every French town and city. It has been stated that American engineers are showing interest in the experiment, which might prove a valuable model in overcoming the difficulties now faced by the United States. The same might surely be said of the United Kingdom.

'The Moon by 1970!' was the call of President Kennedy, spurring on the experts of a nation proud of its technological achievements. With the increasing number of human beings adversely affected by unchecked, uncensored technology, the nation might well have been wiser to listen to the rueful voice of one of its great scientists, Linus Pauling. He had this to say: 'By diverting space dollars, it would be possible to learn one thousand interesting and important things about the human body for one question answered about the moon.' His plea went unheeded. How could the glamour of Man rival that of the Moon?

Not that we in Western Europe can take any pride in the direction of our own technological progress. In his Reith Lectures for 1969, Professor (now Sir) Frank Fraser Darling left us in no doubt that we have sacrificed our environment to this false god, although in his opinion, even at this late hour, we might still save the world from making itself uninhabitable to our species. Therefore, as he sees it, 'The integrity of the environment should be a primary responsibility of any advanced nation.'

Even advanced nations are ruled and directed by governments and industries, however, and these institutions are notoriously slow movers where payments not profits are to be made. To many of us today it seems that the primary responsibility lies on every one of us as individuals. Therefore the essential thing is, in the old Quaker phraseology, to 'have a concern' for the future as well as the present, to care enough to feel personally involved and ready to shoulder that share of the task which lies in our hand, without waiting for rules and penalties compelling us to play a reluctant part. In the words of a great physiologist, the late Sir Charles Sherrington, 'We have, because human, an inalienable prerogative of responsibility which we cannot devolve, no, not as was once thought, even upon the stars. We can share it only with each other.'

INDEX

A. M. A., 122
A. M. A. Arch Path., 121
Abdominal Decompression, a Monograph
(Heynes), 93
Actinotherapy and Diathermy (Clayton), 110
Actions and Uses of Drugs (Sapeika), 93, 110,
122, 184
Advancement of Science, American Association
for the, 170
Aerosols
inflammable content of, 97, 107
pyrethrum, 122
Agron. Jour., 209
Air Around Us, The (Chandler), 43
Air Pollution and Respiratory Diseases
Symposium, New York, 52
Alcohol and Drug Addicts (Treatment) Board,
Adelaide, 140
Alcohol, chemical insecticides and, 121
Alcoholic Psychosis, The (Malzberg), 139
Alcoholics Anonymous, 128, 135–8, 140–1, 149
General Service Board of, New York, 141
Alcoholism, Chapter 8
Co-operative Commission on the Study of,
132
danger of hidden, 124, 126, 134, 138
National Council on, 131–3, 136, 140
psychosomatic disease, 129
vitamin deficiency in, 136
world's biggest public health problem, 124
Alcoholism (Kessel, Walton), 139
Alcoholism, The Disease Concept of (Jellinek),
125, 139
Alcoholism in an English County, A Survey of,
(Moss Davies), 139
Alcoholism in Industry (National Lifeline),
139–40
Alexander, Peter, 64
Alkali Act, 13
Am. J. Clin. Nut., 93–4, 155, 184, 196
Am. Jour. Clin. Path., 33
Am. J. Dig. Dis., 185
Am. Jour. Dis. Chil., 185
Am. J. Hp. Pharm., 93–4
Am. J. Nursing, 94, 122
Am. J. Obst. and Gyn., 93–4
Am. J. Psych., 139
Am. J. Pub. Health, 34
Am. Soc. Heat. & Vent. Engs., 43
Am. Vet. Med. Ass., 122
American Air Transport Association, 48
American Cancer Society, 65, 180, 183
American Dental Association, Journal of the, 63
American Medical Association, 114, 122, 184–5,
194
American Medical Society, 128
Amphetamines, 83–4
Amputation by rotary mower, 109
Anaemia, Vitamin E and, 79
Anaesthes, 93

Ann. Acc. Applied Nutrition, 154
Ann. de la Facul. de Med., 34
Ann. Occup. Hyg., 43
Annals of Allergy, 25, 34, 54
Anns. Int. Med., 209
Ant repellents, safe, 120–1
Antibiotics, toxic exposure from, 85
Anticipations (Wells), 50
Apex Trust, 137
Arch. des Ma. Prof. due Tr. et de S. Soc., 34
Arch. Environ. Health, 33, 43, 53–4
Arch. für Gewerbe p. u. Gewerbehyg., 33
Arch. Mal. Prof., 139
Arch. Za Hig. RADA, 69
Armitage, S. G., 93
Army Medical Research & Nut. Lab. Report, 54
Arteries furred by stop–go dieting, 160
Artificial sweeteners undesirable, 151–2
Arzneimittelforsch, 54
Asphyxia by gas, treatment for, 41
Aspirin, iron deficiency anaemia and, 79
Asst. Gyn. and Obstr. Tutorial, 93
Atheroma, 191–2
Aviation Medicine, RCAF Institute of, 45
Ayres, Robert U., 49

BEAB mark for protection, 106
Babies, passivity unhealthy in, 158
Bacon, Francis, 133
Bailey, Herbert, 94, 154, 184
Baker, H., 155
Banting, F. G., 146
Barbiturates, malathion and, 116
Bartels, H., 93
Basic Principles of Ventilation and Heating
(Bedford), 34, 43
Bauer, H. K., 174, 184
Bear, F. E., 185
Beard, R. R. 34
Beck, Harvey, 34
Bedford, Thomas, 34, 43
Bell, Milton, 33
Bennington, J., 70
Benzopyrenes, lung cancer suspect, 177
Bernardino, R., 34
Bibl. Paediat., 94
Bichel, H., 94
Bicknell, Franklin, 93, 110, 195
Bierstreker, K., 33
Biochem. Journ, 185
Biology and Ethics Symposium, 71
Bio-Science, 111
Biphenyls, polychlorinated, 106
Biskind, Morton, 113, 185
Blackburn, Raymond, 134
Blond, Kaspar, 185
Blood, 185
Board of Trade Business Monitor, 110
Bogert, E. J., 192, 195
Bonfires, cancer from, 109

Book of Poisons, The (Schenk), 33, 121
Boron, 121
Brambell Report, 168
Bread, harmful bleach in white, 80
Bread (Horder, Dodds, Moran), 184–5
Breakfast, importance of cooked, 207–8
Breast milk, high vitamin A content of, 179
Breath of Life, The (Carr), 34, 43, 54
Breuil, M., 34
Brewer's yeast
    for alcoholics, 136–7
    cure for acne, 148
Bridges' Food and Beverage Analyses (Mattice), 154, 184–5, 196
Brinkman, R., 43
Brit. Assoc. for the Advancement of Science, Council of the, 195
Brit. J. Nut., 93
Brit. Med. Bull., 185, 209
British Dental Association, 146
British Empire Cancer Campaign, 171, 179
British Industrial Biological Research Association, 152
British J. Prev. Soc. Med., 70
British Medical Journal, 15 n., 62, 69, 70, 76, 93, 110, 122
British Standards Institution, 29, 31, 34, 37, 108
Brock, J. F., 61
Bronchitis
    prevalence in mining areas, 25
    sulphur dioxide and, 14
    tobacco a correlate of, 56
Burr, G. O., 185
Byrne, Alfred, 93

Cabrini, Dentkos M., 93–4
Callow, A. B., 184
Cameron, Charles S., 185
Cameron, Ewan, 23, 156
Campbell, D. G., 33
Campbell, G. D., 154
Canadian Federation on Alcoholic Problems, Toronto, 141
Canadian Medical Association Journal, 19, 33, 93, 122, 185
Cancer, 70
Cancer
    Congress, Germany, (1954), 174
    defence against, 82
    diet lacking vitamins favours, 174
    in old age, childhood exposure leading to, 183
    Institute, Louvain, 174
    nutrition to fortify body against, 168
    prophylaxis, 174
    protective measures against, 170–3
    result of bad habits, 180–1, 183
    second largest cause of death among children, 170
    whole wheat, riboflavin and, 175
Cancer Research, 184
Cannabis, 86; c. indica, 86
Car exhaust fumes, 17, 44–8
Car sickness, fumes cause of, 53

Carbon-tetra-chloride, 97–8
Carbon monoxide, Chapter 1
    detection, 35–6
    effect in bloodstream, 15
    from cars, 44–8
    indicator, futility of, 46
    intoxication, 11, 19, 22–3
    poisoning, 12, 15–25
    traffic accidents and, 54
Carboxyhaemoglobin, 15, 19–20, 22, 45, 54
Carcinogen, -s,
    dieldrin a, 119
    food additives suspect as, 192
    in food, 173, 175
    nitrous oxide as potential, 47
    saccharine a suspect, 151
    smoking and, 59
    synthetic sweeteners and, 151, 160
    Vitamin A protects against, 177
Carper, Jean, 110
Carr, Donald, 28, 34, 43, 54
Carson, Rachel, 111, 173
Casmey, W. H., 43
Cassidy, W. E., 121
Castle, Barbara, 45, 53, 130
Catalase
    agents destructive to, 181–2
    fundamental defence enzyme, 180
    protective against cancer, 199
Cereal Chemistry, 196
Chandler, T. J., 43
Charcoal, highest carbon monoxide producer, 25
Chemical additives, protection against, 171–2
Chemicals, Humus and the Soil (Hopkins), 195
Chemicals in Food and Farm Produce (Bicknell, Franklin), 93, 110, 195
Chester Beatty Research Institute, 64
Children, keeping household poisons from, 108
Children's Cancer Research Foundation Meeting, (1969), 117
Children's Nightdress Regulations (1964), 107
Chlorinated hydrocarbon, 96, 181
Chlorine dioxide, 80
Chlorine gas from lavatory cleansers, 96
Chromosomes, drug damage to, 86
Chronic CO Poisoning (Grut), 33
Churchill, John A., 194, 196
Circle Trust, 137–8
Clarke, I., 185
Clayton, E. C., 110
Clean Air Act, 13, 37, 173
Cleave, C. T., 154
Clinical Toxicology of Commercial Products (Gleason), 110, 119, 122, 196
CO and Chronic CO Poisoning (Raymond, Vallaud), 34
Coal fire, correct feeding of, 36
cockroaches, repelling, 121
Cohen of Birkenhead, Lord, 55
Coke and Gas (Minchin), 33
Coke fumes, 12–14
Cold Harbour Laboratory of Quantitive Biology, 172 n.
Committee on Toxicology, 122
Commoner, Barry, 50

Complete Slimmer, The (Yudkin), 167
Congenital Malformations, International Conference on, 89
Consumer Reports, 155
Consumers Association, 103, 115
Contraception, 72
Cook, responsibility of, 197–8
    trade marks of good, 198
Cooking and Nutritive Value (Callow), 184
Coronary thrombosis, sugar and, 145
Council of Europe, 212–13
Council on Pharmacy and Chemistry, 122
Craig, J. Oman, 159
Cyclamates, 152, 160
    research findings awaited, 160
    Ministry of Agriculture bans, 152
Cycle of Life, The (film), 195

DDT, 111–14, 181
    banned, 113
    contradictory views on, 112–14
    poisoning, symptoms of, 113
DNA molecule, 172
Dale, W. E., 121
Daniel, Esther, 184
Darling, Sir Frank Fraser, 214
Davies, E. Beresford, 139
Davis, Adelle, 164, 167, 198, 205
Davis, Dorothy V., 110
Davy, John, 212
De Go, Pierre Marie, 134
Debré, Robert, 127
Decorating, dangers in do-it-yourself, 106
Denture cleansers, toxic, 96
Deodorants, harmful, 95
Dermatology, Hallamshire Hospital, Department of, 103–4
Desrosier, N. W., 209
Detergent danger, 101–2, 173
Diabetes, Coronary Thrombosis and the Saccharine Diseases (Cleave, Campbell), 144, 154
Diabetes, large babies and maternal, 158
Dichlorvos, 114, 117
Dieldrin, 118–19, 181
Diet
    arteries furred by, 160
    cholesterol balance disturbed by stop–go, 160
    items in a balanced, 187
    no better therapy than well-balanced, 194
    supplementing deficient, 209–10
Dietetics Simplified (Bogert), 195
Dimbleby, Richard, 170
Direction of Human Development, The, (Montagu), 34
Diseases of the Chest, Institute of, 54
Ditchburn, R. W., 185
Doctor training, low emphasis on prevention, 210–11
Dodds, C., 184–5
Doll, R., 64, 70, 84
Draught excluders, dangers of, 30, 37
Driesbach, Robert H., 33, 93, 122
Drinking and Alcoholism (Kemp), 139
Drummond, Sir Jack, 151, 193

Dry cleaning, harmful fumes from, 98–100
Duddington, C. L., 162, 166
Dyle, C. E., 122

Early Diagnosis of Anaemia, The, (Kilpatrick), 93
Edison, Thomas Alva, 50
Egler, F. E., 111, 121
Eisenhower, Dwight D., 60
Electric car
    feasible, 51–3
    vested interests against, 50, 173
    virtues of, 50–1
Electric light, no future for, 50, 52
Electricity, least unhealthy, 12, 36
Elizabeth I, 35, 120, 143
Elvejhem, C. A., 184
Elwood, P. C., 80, 93
Endocrinology, 185
Enzymes in detergents, perils of, 103
European Conservation Conference, Strasbourg, 48, 212
European Conservation Year. United Kingdom. 1970 (Nature Conservancy), 212
Exercise
    for abdominal muscles, 165–6
    mother-to-be and, 90

Fels Institute, Yellow Springs, 91
Females the fat sex, 159
Fertilizers, artificial, 188–9
Fire accidents in home, 107–8
Fish
    more wholesome than meat, 206
    ways of cooking, 206–7
Fit for Life (Beric Wright), 210
Fitzhugh, Garth O., 93
Flour, inadequate extraction rate in white, 175
Flues, relining of, 38
Fluoridation, 146, 181
Fluoride, cumulative catalase poison, 181
Foam, futility of, 102
Fol. Med., 34
Food
    and Drug Administration (USA), 85, 97
    and Drug, Association of, 115
    denatured, 88
    experts' list of perfectly constituted, 187
    Hygiene Regulations (1956), 114
    refining, vitamin deficiency and, 192
Food and Cosmetics Toxicology, 121
Food and Nutrition (AMA), Council for, 187, 195
Food Facts and Fallacies (Fredericks, Bailey), 94, 154, 184
Food Science & Technology (Pyke), 195
Food Trade Review, 122
Forbes, J. C., 139
France, world's highest alcoholic rate, 126
Fredericks, Carlton, 94, 143, 154, 184
Frederickson, Donald, 61
Freiburg Gynaecological Clinic, 77
Fruit
    for sweet-toothed, cooking, 149
    raw, 199
    rules for keeping nutrition in, 200–1

Frying pan, toxicity with non-stick, 105
Fuerst, Harold T., 18

Gardening, danger areas in, 108–9
Gas, dangers with domestic, 25–32
Gas Act (1948), 37
Gerstley, J. R., 154
'Getting Married' (Trimmer), 144
Gigiena i Sanitariya, 122
Gilbert, F. A., 192, 195
Glasgow Council on Alcoholism, 140
Gleason, M. N., 110, 122, 196
Gluconate, ferrous, 80
Glucose, harmful commercial, 151
Glycogen, 145
Godber, Sir George, 55–6, 64
Goodhart, H. S., 185
Gould, Donald, 66
Gout from beer, 130
Grace, E. J., 65
Grant, Doris, 176
Gray, C. H., 110
Gruen, L., 43
Gruenwald, P., 33
Grut, A., 21, 33
Guide to Parasitology (Blackwell, Southwell), 209
Gundry, Elizabeth, 110

Haddow, Alexander, 62
Haemoglobin, 15, 21–2
Hair lacquer, inflammable, 97
Haldane, J. B. S., 11, 148
Hale, Fred, 87, 94
Hand, D. B., 185
Handbook of Poisoning (Driesbach), 33, 93, 114, 122
Harris, R. J. C., 56, 69
Harwell Atomic Station, 67
Hayes, Wayland, 118, 122
Health and Education, Handbook of, (HMSO), 187, 195
Health Education Journal, 69
Helping Hand Organization, 137
Hepatitis, 16
Heroin, congenital addicition, 86
Heynes, Ockert, 75, 93
Hill, Bradford, 64, 70
Hills, J. B. G., 33–4, 43, 110
Hirschhorn, K, 94
Hollingsworth, D., 195
Hollins, Arthur, 191
Holman, R. A., 185
Honey, high calorie content, 149
Hopkins, Donald, 195
Horder, Lord, 184–5
Horwitt, M. K., 184
Hosp. Management, 69
House into Home, (Kendall), 155
Household hazards, 95–109
Housewives Beware (Grant), 176
Hueper, W. C., 119, 122, 170, 173, 183–5
Hueter, F. G., 54
Hull, G. W., 195
Hunger to Come, The (Laffin), 153, 155
Huxley, Aldous, 86

Huxley, Elspeth, 144
Hydrocarbons, chlorinated, 111
Hydrogen sulphide, 12, 26

I am an Alcoholic (Blackburn), 134
Imperial Cancer Relief Fund, 171
Imperial Cancer Research Institute, 56
In Place of Poisons (Henry Doubleday Research Association), 123
Ind. Jour. of Med. Res., 196
Ind. Med. and Surgery, 121
Indigestion mixture, riboflavin intake reduced by, 177
Indust. and Engin. Chem., 184
Infants
    fatness undesirable in, 156, 158
    obese, 155
    overfed, 156
Insecticides
    alcohol and chemical, 121
    dangers to humans, 111
    immunized, 111
Inter. Congress Vit. E., 93
Int. Jour. Air Pollution, 33
Internal combustion engine, monarchy of, 173
International Biological Programme, 212
International Cancer Congress, Tokyo, (1966), 177

J.A.M.A., 184–5
J. Am. Diet. Assn., 209
J. Appl. Nut., 184
J. Biol. Chem., 93–4, 184
J. Comp. and Physiol. Psych., 93
J. Nut., 184–5
J. Pediat., 154
Jackson, Joan K., 139
Jellinek, E. M., 125, 139
Jenson, N. E., 110
Johnson, L. B., 60
Johnson, Samuel, 62, 150, 162
Johnston, Lennox, 67
Joliffe, N., 184
Jones, D., 195
Jones, R. J., 185
Josephs, H. W., 185
Joules, H., 69
Jour. Agri. Res., 209
Jour. Am. Med. Assoc., 69, 122
Jour. Dental Res., 93
Jour. Digest. Disturb., 33
Jour. of Medical. Sci., 43
Jour. of Phar. and Exp. Therap., 121
Jour. Soil Assoc., 93, 185, 195
Journal of RoSPA, 110

Kailin, E. W., 122
Katz, M., 33
Keep it Clean (Low), 110
Kemp, Robert, 139, 157
Kench, J. E., 44, 54
Kendall, Elizabeth, 155
Kennedy, J. F., 214
Kensler, C. J., 184
Keonig, Oskar, 195

Kershbaum, A., 69
Kessel, Neil, 139
Kilgore, L., 196, 209
Kilpatrick, G. S., 93
Kimble, M. S., 184
Kimmey, James, 130
Kingsley, Charles, 72
Kiss of life, 41
Kitchen, ventilation of, 26, 28
Klein, L., 110
Klenner, F., 185
Kolbuszewski, J., 52
Krebsproblem, Das (Bauer), 174, 184
Kreshoven, S. J., 93
Kreuta, M., 185
Kushner, D. S., 94

LSD, 85-6
Laboratory Handbook of Toxic Agents (Gray, ed.), 110
Laffin, John, 153, 155
Lancet, 43, 70, 80, 93-4, 160, 166, 184, 195
Laug, E P., 121
Lawrence, J. M., 196
Lead poisoning from toiletry, 96-7
Lear, John, 171
Lear, William, 49
Lebon, Phillip, 159
Leçons de Toxicologie (Raymond, Vallaud), 33
Lee, Fred, 26
Lemere, F., 139
Let's Get Well (Davis), 167
Leukaemia, LSD and, 86
Leukocytosis, 19
Lewis, B., 195
Liddicoat, Renée, 93
Liebig, Justus, 189
Life Before Birth (Montagu), 69, 93-4
Lindane, 114-16
    high toxicity, 115
    used in paints, 115
Lindgren, D. L., 122
Linklater, Eric, 183
Liquid paraffin
    condemned by American Medical Association, 179
    harmful, 80, 88
    robber of Vitamin A, 178-9
Little, W. A., 94, 122
Liver and Cancer, The (Blond), 185
Liver in Circulatory Diseases, The (Sherlock), 33
Living Brain, The (Walter), 94
Lloyd, F. T., 69
Loew, O., 185
Lofroth, Goran, 117, 119, 122, 212
London Alcoholism Information Centre, The, 140
Los Angeles County Air Pollution Control Laboratory, 46
Los Angeles Times, 143
Low, Lia, 110
Lowe, C. R., 93
Lowell, Philip M., 143
Lung cancer, smoking a correlate of, 56
Lurie, J. B., 122

Maenpaa, P. H., 139
McCarrison, Sir Robert, 143, 186-9, 192-6
McCollum, E. V., 209
McCurdy, Robert, 69
Macfarland, Ross A., 54
McGraw Encyclopedia of Science and Technology, The, 110
MacNamara, W. D., 54
Magnesium pemoline, 23
Maier-Bode, H., 122
Maisin, J., 174, 184
Malathion, 116-17
Mallach, H. J., 54
Malzberg, B., 139
Man Against Himself (Menninger), 139
Manchester Univ. Med. School Gazette, 54
Mann, H., 70
Manual of Nutrition, (HMSO), 184
Maranzana, P., 33
Martin, W. C., 184
Masai Story, The (Keonig), 195
Mathill, H. A., 93
Mattice, M. R., 154, 184-5, 196
Meat, molasses to increase supply, 154
Meatless diet, care in choice of, 206
Med. Annals Dis. Columbia, 122
Med. Exp., 122
Med. Zn. Uzbek USSR, 34
Medical Information Service, Munich, 40
Medical Jour. of Australia, 139
Medical News, 196
Medical Officer, 69, 131
Medical Press and Circular, 189, 195
Medical Services Journal, Canada, 45, 54
Melchior, J. C., 93
Mendès-France, Pierre, 126
Menninger, William, 139
Mental Health, National Institute of, 130
'Metabolism, congenital errors of', 88
Metropolitan Transport Authority, 52
Mey, R., 93
Michelson, O., 184
Micro-organisms as Allies (Duddington), 166
Miller, Z., 94
Mills, C. A., 39, 43
Minchin, L. T., 33
Minerva Medica, 33
Mineral Nutrition and the Balance of Life (Gilbert), 195
Ministry of Labour Gazette (HMSO), 144, 154
Misrahy, G. A., 93
Mitford, Nancy, 171
Modern Nutrition in Health and Disease (Wohl, Goodhart), 185
Montagu, Ashley, 24, 34, 69, 72, 74, 93-4
Month. Bull. Min. H and Pub. Health Lab. Service, 121-2
Moore, T., 185
Moran, T., 184-5
Morant, D., 196
Moss, M. C., 139
Mothers-to-be, advice for, 91
Mothproofing, danger from, 119
Moths, safe action against, 119-20
Motoyama, E. K., 94

Munch. Med. Wocksehr, 43, 93
Municipal Engineering, 34
Murphy, D. P., 94
Murphy, S. E., 122
Murray, Middleton, 72

N.Y. Acad. of Science, 185
Narcotics, UN Commission on, 86, 94
National Audubon Society, 113
National Cancer Institute, USA, The, 170
National Coal Board, 13
National Council on Alcoholism
    Johannesburg, 141
    New York, 141
National Lifeline, 137
National Poisons Information Service, 194
National Research Council (USA), 152
National Society of Cancer Relief, 171, 184
National Society on Alcoholism, Wellington, 141
National Society for Clean Air, 51
Nature, 110, 155, 185, 195
New Domestic Encyclopedia (Davis), 110
New Eng. J. Med., 184
New Orleans Med. & Surg. Jour., 34
New Scientist, 27, 54, 93, 94, 117, 122, 154, 155, 172, 179, 185
New York Academy of Sciences, 63
New York State Jour. Med., 94
Nicholson, Max, 212
Nitrates dangerous for babies, 200
Nitrous oxides, 32, 39, 47
Non-Smokers, National Society of, 58, 68
Nose desensitized to perfumed propellants, 96
Not to Frighten but to Enlighten (National Society for Cancer Relief), 184
Nursing Outlook, 93
Nuts. Abs. and Revs. 185, 196
Nut. Ac. Sci. Nat. Res. Council, 154
Nut. Review, 93, 185
Nutrients to combat obesity, 161
Nutrition and Health (McCarrison), 195
Nutrition
    faulty food upsets function of, 187
    lifetime study of, 186
Nutritional Values in Crops and Plants (Schuphan), 209

Obesity, 156–60
    foods causing, 157
    heart failure and, 157
    in middle age, 157
    overeating the cause of, 157
    starving no cure for, 160
Obesity Association, 159
Observer, The, 115, 196
Oettingen, W. F., 17
Ogilvy, Sir Heneage, 174, 181
Ohio State Med. J., 185
Oil Heater Regulations (1963), 32
Oil heaters, noxious fumes from, 32–3, 37
'On the State of Public Health' (HMSO), 69
Orent-Keiles, E., 209
Oreston, T. R., 155
Organo-chlorines, 111, 115–16, 119–20, 122–3

Organo-phosphates, 115–18, 122–3, 194
Ortega, P., 121
Overweight, more women than men, 159
Overweight Society, The (Wyden), 156, 166
Oxygen
    deficiency, 15–24, 41, 55, 83
    under pressure as resuscitant, 40
    vital prenatal need for, 73–6
Ozone
    an irritant, 39
    toxicity, 39–40, 47

Para-di-chloro-benzene, 95, 181
Paraffin, lethal fumes from, 32–3
Paraffin liquid, 80, 88, 178–9
Parasites, cooking destroys, 199
Parkes, Sir Alan, 71
Pauling, Linus, 214
Peacock, P. R., 185, 209
Peas, colouring in processed, 200
Pecora, L., 34
Peden, J. D., 122
Per-chloroethylene, 98
Perelli, G., 33
Pesticide -s,
    residues, 111, 173, 194
    Government advisory committee on, 113
    pets and dermatitis, 117–18
    profit motive and, 111
Petry, A., 33
Pfeiffer, Ehrenfried, 181, 189, 195
Philip, Prince, 46, 212
Phillips, William, 156
Phys. Rev., 185
Pill, the, 72, 84–5
Pillemer, L. A., 185
Platt, Lord, 61
Playpen
    encourages premature standing, 158
    prevents development, 158
Poison in air, 11–33
Polchenko, V. I., 122
Polystyrene tiles, fire risk of, 107
Post Office Research Station, Dollis Hill, 12
Potassium Symposium, 185
Potato crisps, double calorie content in, 157
Potatoes, vitamin source, 157
Power Sources Symposium, Sixth International, 52
Practitioner, The, 139, 157
Praxidoxine, 194
Premature birth, 74
Prevention of Cancer, The (Raven, Roe, eds.), 168, 173, 199, 209
Price, Weston, 148, 154
Proc. Nut. Soc., 195
Proc. Am. Assoc. for Cancer Research, 185
Proc. Am. Soil Sci. Soc., 185
Proc. Royal Society, 122
Proc. Roy. Soc. of Med., 33
Proc. Soc. Exp. Biol. and Med., 122, 195
Proc. U.S. Nat. Acad. Science, 139
Protection of the Environment—the fight against pollution, The (HMSO), 211
Proteinuria, 19

Public Health Reports Supplement (National Cancer Institute), 122, 184
Public Transport Association, 52
Pyke, Magnus, 195
Pyrethrum for insect control, 116

Quart. Jour. of Studies on Alcohol, 139
Quarterly Bulletin, 115

R. J. Appl. Nut., 185
Radford, E. P., Jr., 93
Radomski, J. L., 121
Rancidity in Oils (Townsend), 185
Ransom, B. H., 209
Rassegna de Medicina Indust., 33
Raven, Ronald, 66, 168, 199, 209
Raventros, A., 94
Raymond, V., 33, 34, 139
Re-crystallization substance, danger in use, 115
Red Strangers (Huxley), 144
Reid, Lynne, 54, 69
Reilly, K. A., 139
Reisman, K. R., 185
Relaxation, 81–3
Residues Review, 122
Rev. Belg. des Sciences Medicales, 184
Rev. Cubana Cienc. Agric., 155
Rhoads, C. P., 185
Riboflavin
    destroyed in kitchen, 176
    fundamental defence vitamin against cancer, 174
    indigestion mixtures reduce, 177
    simple way of obtaining, 176
    sources of, 177
    whole wheat and, 175
Rimington, J., 70
River Pollution (Klein), 110
Road Traffic Conference, Vienna, Third International, 51
Roberts, Goronwy, 48
Roberts, W. A. B., 93
Rodale, J. I., 162
Rose, F. J. C., 169, 199, 209
Roskill Commission, 51
Royal Cancer Hospital, 66
Royal College of Physicians, 61
Royal Society for the Prevention of Accidents, 29, 43, 97, 107–8
Russell, C. S., 77, 93

S. Afr. Med. J., 93
Saccharine, carcinogen suspect, 151
Safety Precautions Scheme, UK Pesticide, 117
Saffiotti, U., 177
Salad
    all the year, 202
    definition of, 201
    virtues of, 201
Sangster, J. F., 69
Santayana, George, 189

Sapeika, N., 93, 110, 122, 184
Saturday Review, 172
Schenk, Gustav, 16, 33, 121
Schilling, Richard, 104
Schlachter, S., 167
Schrimshaw, N. S., 209
Schuphan, W., 200, 209
Schutte, K. H., 195
Science, 94, 121–2, 167, 184
Science Journal, 110
Science Newsletter, 33
Sequiera, Dr, 89
Shapiro, S., 185
Sharman, L. M., 93
Sherman, H. C., 162
Sheff. Univ. Gazette, 93
Sherrington, Sir Charles, 215
Sherlock, Sheila, 33
Shop and Railway Premises Act (1963), 29 n
Shils, M. E., 94
Shute, Evan, 88, 94
Silent Spring (Carson), 113, 173
Slimming
    adults and, 156
    garments, waste of money, 161
    pills dangerous, 161
Smith, Alan, 13, 33
Smith, J., 122
Smoking and Health, New York, World Conference on, 65
Smoking and Health, Report by Royal College of Physicians, 70
Smoking
    filter fallacy, 61
    harmful to others, 56–7
    lettuce leaf, 62
    personality traits, 63–4
    pregnancy and, 58, 63, 74, 76–8
    the Pill and, 84–5
Smoking, Lung Cancer and You (McCurdy), 69
Smolyask, M., 34
Snuff, 62–3
Snuff Grinders, Blenders, Purveyors and Connoisseurs, Society of, 62
Soap
    safety in, 100–1, 104–5
    water softeners to aid, 105
Soft Drink Regulations (1964), 160
Soil Association Haughley Experiment, 195
Soil Conservation Department, FAO, 210
Soil Crop Science Soc., Florida, 185
Soil fertility, decline in, 187–8
Soil Fertility, Renewal and Preservation (Pfeiffer), 195
Soil, Grass and Cancer (Voisin), 179, 184–5
South African Industrial Chemist, 155
Southern Med. Jour., 185
Speizer, F. E., 33
Spencer, T. D., 43
Stain removers, toxic, 100
Stamp, Dudley, 189, 195
State Research Laboratory, Helsinki, 129
Stay Alive (Carpenter, Gundry), 110
Steam cf. petrol, 49

Stewart, William, 64
Stokinger, H. E., 39, 43
Stuart-Harris, C. H., 110
Stubbs, Peter, 172
Sucrose, real term for refined sugar waste, 144–5
Sugar
  abolition substitute for dentistry, 146
  addiction to, 142
  alternatives, 149
  cane, natural goodness in, 143
  cane waste, humans buy, 144
  cane waste, newsprint from, 153
  enemy of health, 145
  growing, alternatives to, 152–4
  ills from, 142
  industrial alternatives, 153–4
  into detergents, 153
  low blood, 150
  refining a robbery, 143–4
  robber of vitamins, 143–4
  substitutes harmful, 151–2
  'The Great White Lie', 143
Sulphur dioxide, 12–14, 26–7, 38
Sunday Times, 37, 93
Sweet tooth a curse, 142
Sweeteners suspected carcinogens, synthetic, 160
Sweets, combating effect of eating, 149–50
Swell, L., 195
Sykes, Friend, 191
Synthetic Detergents, Report of the Committee on (HMSO), 110
Syphilis, treatment of unborn children, 89

Taylor, W. J. R., 122
Taylor, Geoffrey, 193, 196
Technology of Food Preservation, The (Desrosier), 209
Tedeschi, C. G., 93
Teenagers, increased alcoholism among, 125
Temperature inversion, 46
Tenancy above dry cleaners, 99–100
Tension, relief from, 80–3
Ternisien, Jean, 214
Tetraethyl lead, 97
Texas Agricultural Experimental Station, 87
Texas S. J. Med., 94
Thalidomide, 78, 89
Thermo Electron Corporation, 49
Theron, Randolph, 25, 34, 54
Thompson, M. M., 93, 155
Thomson, William, 93
Thorn, G. W., 209
Tobacco, tax receipts from, 55
Toilet preparations, hazardous, 96–7
Townsend, G. O., 185
Tranquillizers, 80–1, 83
Tri-chloro-ethylene, 97–8
Trichlorphon, 120
Trimmer, Eric, 144
Tropical Products Institute, London, 153
Truth about Cancer, The (Cameron), 185
Turner, Newman, 191
TV sets, combustible, 107

Univ. of Freiburg Gyn. Med. Klin., 93
US Dept. of Agric. Circular, 209
US Dept. of Agric. Rept. No. 68, 185
Utensils, selection of domestic, 105–6

Valic, F., 69
Vallaud, A., 31, 33–4
Vallaud, E. V., 139
Van Raalte, H. G. S., 121
Vaporizers, electric, 114–15, 117
Vedder, P. B., 185
Vegetables
  boiling bad for, 204
  raw, 198–9
  rules for preserving nutrition in, 200–1
Ventilation, gas and, 26, 28, 30–1, 37
Verzar, F., 93
Vessey, M. P., 84
Vit. E. Symposium Ann., 94
Vitamin A
  robbers of, 178–9
  sources, 178
Vitamin B complex depletion, 89–90
Vitamin C, sources of, 177 n.
Vitamin deficiency, 175, 193–4
Voisin, André, 174, 179, 184–5
Von Post-Lingin, M. L., 33

Waddell, J., 93
Walsh, T., 185
Walter, W. Grey, 91, 94
Walton, Henry, 199
Walton, Isaak, 208
Watson, John D., 172 n.
Way to the Smokeless City, The (Casmey), 43
Welles, Orson, 161
Wells, H. G., 50
Westlake, Aubrey, 93
What You Should Know about Tobacco (Wood), 69
Which?, 115
White, P. L., 195
Whitehead, A. N., 151
Wholemeal flour, 175, 208
Wigglesworth, Dr, 195
Wilde, Oscar, 16
Williams, H. J., 184
Williams, Lincoln, 133, 139
Williams, Roger J., 128–9, 139, 184
Willemse, A. G. S., 122
Willis, G. C., 185
Wilson, J. W., 209
Winninck, Myron, 93
Wise, R. C., 185
Witheridge, W. N., 43
Wohl, M. G., 185
Woollens, dieldrin in, 119
Women ban noxious fumes, 35
Wood, F. L., 56, 69
World Health Assembly, Geneva, 23rd, 210
World Health Organization, 117–18, 122, 125, 137, 209
World weight record, 156
Wright, H. Beric, 210
Wryden, Peter, 156, 166

X-ray, pregnancy test before, 85
Xylene hazardous to user, 100, 106

Yearbook Separate No. 1681 (US Dept. Agric.), 184
Yeast, brewer's, 84–5, 136–7, 148, 161

Yeast from sugar, 153
Yerby, Alonso S., 94
Yudkin, John, 142, 145, 167

Zaffi, Juan, 182, 185